Zen and the Art of Giving
up Smoking
and Vaping

ZEN AND THE ART OF GIVING UP SMOKING AND VAPING

FootSteps Press First Edition
www.footstepsbooks.com

Cover Design © Basia Bird

Illustrations by Nick Holden and Basia Bird

ISBN 978-1-908867-98-8

Zen and the Art of Giving up Smoking and Vaping

by

Nick Holden

Special thanks to:
David Lambert, Jessica Woolard,
Anna Caldwell, Jane Graham-Maw

CHAPTERS

1

INTRODUCTION

This book was born out of an epiphany. A single moment of self-realization, beyond which my life was forever changed. But that single moment was born out of a whole cultural period during which a multitude of events, conversations, observations and realizations all coalesced in a perfect moment of truth.

I was a smoker, and then I wasn't.

And that was just the beginning, in more ways than I could have imagined.

The time was the 1990s; the culture was the British electronic dance scene. A time of underground parties, repetitive beats, psychedelic drugs and social liberation. As a creative movement, it sharply polarised society, giving birth both to legislation that sought to suppress it, and a worldwide creative influence that was unprecedented in its reach. For those of us swept along by its tide, it was an incredibly exciting time. It appeared on the surface to be a hedonistic movement, and for certain this was part of the picture. But equally there was a sense of something both ancient and tribal being rediscovered, and something futuristic and evolutionary unfolding from within.

The prevalence of psychoactive substances, over the more rudimentary intoxicants of mainstream culture, fostered a receptivity, and a genuine climate of self-exploration. In the after-hours beyond the dance floor, people debated existential questions, and there was a real sense that answers were hanging in the air, ready to be plucked and held to light. The prevailing atmosphere felt pregnant with possibility.

For many such as me, the culture encompassed all facets of life, from income to social networks to entertainment, and, gradually, an emerging sense of spiritual awareness that ultimately directed my focus to the East.

After the realization that ended my nicotine addiction, I felt as though I had passed into a parallel world, in which smoking was no longer the supportive companion that I had taken it for. **I had understood that nicotine was in fact the source of the problem I had thought I was using it to solve**. I felt like Alice, through the looking glass, never to return. I was living in a world that whilst it appeared essentially the same, was in one major respect, the reverse image of the one I had left behind. I started to share what I had experienced, with a proactive compulsion, and quickly discovered that I had an aptitude for communicating my experience, and thus began guiding others through the same portal.

In those after-hours times, I took on the role of "the guy who can help you stop smoking", who if you sought him out, and found him in the appropriate mood, would talk you out of your addiction, so that it left you free to begin a new, healthier, less stressful, life as a non-smoker. Sometimes this would take merely minutes, as I would sense a specific connection occur, and know, as surely as if I were assembling a familiar jigsaw, that within a few carefully chosen sentences the person I was talking to would without doubt move irreversibly beyond their addiction.

What I didn't anticipate, however, was how this situation would evolve, both for myself and others. The conscious mechanism behind my realization continued to work on a subconscious level, actuated by the lucidity of a mind newly liberated from the shackles of dependency. The perceptual lens through which I had apprehended the nature of my addiction, not only remained open, but over the coming months and years, came to inform my whole state of consciousness. There is more to truly transcending an addiction, than simply the immediate result. The conscious mechanism behind the comprehension process is fundamental to the development of the self. It is the very heart of realization, the primal moment of the acquisition of new seed-level information, that precipitates transformation to a higher state of consciousness. The epiphany that liberated me from nicotine, recalibrated and upgraded my entire cognitive faculty. Over the coming period, this gradually brought me to a succession of spiritual realizations that changed my life almost beyond recognition. As time has passed and my spiritual practice has deepened, I have come to observe a correlation between this journey out of addiction, and core concepts of many of the world's great spiritual traditions. The epiphany that I experienced, and have observed in others who have been through the same process, might be compared to a moment of Satori, or Kensho – seeing one's original face, one's true nature. A momentary return to a state of innocence and purity, within which the addiction has no agency, and from which the seeds of transformation may grow.

This is a unique point in history, and the commercial tobacco/e-cigarette industries are phenomena specific to this time, as is the synthesis and commercial use of nicotine. Despite shifts and evolutions in the manner of its consumption, and a decline in smoking in some parts of the world, the drug maintains a vast grip on the population, and despite widespread awareness of the health issues, enjoys a morally questionable level of cultural acceptance. The commercial tobacco industry remains one of the largest industries on the planet, and one of the primary causes of death to our species. And now under the guise of a "healthier alternative", the vaping industry has expanded with exponential pace, especially through the younger population. Given this ubiquity, it seems reasonable that this phenomenon might conceivably yield something of value for us to learn. As children, from the point at which we first begin to form an impression of the world, we are exposed to the concept of smoking. It is a truly global phenomenon, and even if we have no interest in pursuing it, by-and-large we accept its presence, and will have formed some idea of what it constitutes. On this level, then, the subtle indoctrination that lays the foundations of nicotine addiction, is occurring from very early in life, simply in terms of a basic acceptance of it as a valid aspect of the world as we perceive it. In a sense, a return to who we were in that earlier phase of life, before this process even began, is key to transcending the addiction; and by extension the addiction itself, in its unravelling, is a key to understanding ourselves. We need to bridge the schism in our nature, created by nicotine addiction. We need to reconnect with our original self, and from that perspective, re-evaluate who we have become in the present. We need to reconnect with our essential nature and become whole again. We need to remember our unadulterated wholeness. This is what we are working with here. This begins with smoking, but it extends far beyond the smoking phenomenon, into a path towards self-realization and our higher nature.

At this early point in the journey, I must pay respect to the cultures of the American continent who revere the tobacco plant as sacred. One might deduce from my tone throughout the book, that I have a dislike of tobacco. This is not the case. I have a great respect for this plant, as befits the enormity of its influence, and I feel that it carries a lesson of incredible significance, albeit one that has yet to be widely embraced. It should be noted that in ceremonial use of tobacco amongst these cultures, although it is 'smoked' in a pipe, the smoke is strictly not inhaled, so the relationship is completely different. Even in its original sacred use, tobacco, and by extension its active ingredient nicotine, is not meant to be inhaled. It is the abusive use of the plant in the context of the commercial tobacco and nicotine industries, that I take issue with, and am referring to here.

2

REGARDING THE TITLE

To quote Robert Pirsig, author of *Zen and the Art of Motorcycle Maintenance*, this book "should in no way be associated with that great body of factual information relating to orthodox Zen Buddhist practice" That said, I do feel it is reasonable to associate this book, albeit loosely, with both *Zen in the Art of Archery*, and *Zen and the Art of Motorcycle Maintenance.*

Pirsig's book centres on a motorcycle journey undertaken by himself and his son, accompanied for some of the way by two close friends. This is really just the frame on which he hangs a philosophical essay, in which he both writes in the first person, and also gives form to certain aspects of himself as an independent individual known as Phaedrus. In a similar fashion, it might be said that this book is at its heart an essay on a path to a higher state of consciousness, through the medium of nicotine addiction, albeit in a somewhat lateral fashion. Pirsig's treatment of the self as two distinct personalities, and the relationship between the two, is also a model that I will explore in these pages; namely the pure original self, and the addicted self. Our observations of the disparity between these two aspects of our consciousness, is what will reunite us with our pure nature, and pave the way to a brighter future beyond nicotine addiction.

In the book that was the genesis of this particular nomenclatural grouping, Eugen Herrigel discusses his many years studying archery in Japan, under the Master Awa Kenzô. Herrigel was offered a job teaching philosophy in Japan. He had an interest in Zen, and took the job in part because he felt it represented an opportunity to learn more about it. On seeking tuition in Zen, he was directed to study archery as a precursor to more advanced spiritual practice. This was part of a wider tradition around learning certain motor skills as a way to embrace some of the disposition of Zen. Herrigel studied for several years, and in the book, gives detailed accounts of the technical minutiae of Japanese archery. It is revealed as the book progresses, however, that this detailed and thorough practice is also ultimately leading to a point where the relationship with the art is so advanced, that the sense of the self actually 'doing' anything proactively, dissolves, as do the boundaries between archer and bow, bow and arrow, and Master and disciple. The archer has reached a state of oneness, wherein thoughts of premeditated action disappear, and the arrow shoots itself, the archer simply being part of the interconnected field of Buddha Nature within which this and all things occur. Master Kenzô describes this beautifully:

'Stop thinking about the shot; that way it is

bound to fail. You only feel it because you haven't really let go of your self. It is all so simple. You can learn from an ordinary bamboo leaf, what ought to happen. It bends lower and lower, under the weight of snow. Suddenly the snow slips to the ground without the leaf having stirred. Remain like that, at the point of highest tension, until the shot falls from you. When the tension is fulfilled, the shot must fall. It must fall from the archer, like snow from a bamboo leaf, before the archer even thinks of it.'

This whole progression, from circular observation, through acquisition of awareness, to surrender of the self to higher guidance, leading to a transformative moment of release and change of state – stasis to motion, and conclusion – this is the exact model for the assimilation of the truth that lies in these pages. This is not archery, or Zen, but there is an intriguing similitude between the process we will undertake here, and that undertaken by Herrigel.

What more of a creative art is there, than that of the journey of the self?

The journey back to the original self, our destination beyond the veil of attachment to false realities. The very evolution of consciousness in motion. This is the opportunity that lies within the illusion of nicotine addiction. This is a route to a higher plane. But to get there you must study. Focus, observe, assimilate, understand, to the point that you forget the need to understand, because without even noticing, you have comprehended absolutely, and in so doing are standing in the shoes of the person you always were, looking through the eyes of creation at the simple truth at the heart of it all. You need 'do' no thing at all, besides read, as slowly and carefully as you can, and seek to discern every nuance of what is presented to you.

So to conclude, this is not a Zen text, and I am not a Zen scholar, but I submit that its claim to its title holds merit. Interestingly however, this is in no way by my own design. The title came to me absolutely out of the blue. I wasn't even trying to think of a title at the time. It fell into my awareness like the first flake of snow on a bamboo leaf. I neither sought it nor saw it coming. But it instantly rang true and made me laugh, and further rumination upon the idea brought me to the comparisons I have detailed above. The similarities were there, and the title brought them into view. And this serendipitous occurrence is probably the most Zen aspect of the story of how this book came to be!

3

BEGINNER'S MIND

"In the beginner's mind there are many
possibilities, but in the expert's there are few"
Shunryu Suzuki

People often regard attempts at giving up smoking with a sense of dread. The truth however, is that overcoming nicotine addiction represents a rare opportunity of wondrous proportions, and so should more appropriately be approached with sense of excitement. Rather than thinking about giving up smoking, think more in terms of transcending nicotine addiction. Transcendence means to go beyond one's normal state. In this instance, sadly, 'normality' as we must consider it, is the reality of the addict. To transcend nicotine addiction, a cycle of perception must come to an end, moving you beyond the conceptual sphere of smoking or vaping altogether. On one level you are simply going to rid yourself of a nasty habit, but on another you are embarking on an adventure into uncharted regions of the self. Do not underestimate what a genuinely transformative journey this can be.

Undertaking the process of transcending your nicotine addiction represents an opportunity not just to become healthier, to rid oneself of a bad habit, but to also proactively foster your own conscious evolution. Opportunities this significant do not come along every day! You can beat your addiction. Even if it seems difficult, it does not necessarily follow that it is impossible. The fact is that given the correct approach, it is not especially difficult to beat nicotine addiction. The only real difficulty lies in becoming aware of the correct approach as opposed to the incorrect one, which is where this book comes in.

The first step is to embrace and even to savour the challenge.

My purpose in this book is to help you to unravel the conscious mechanism that lies behind nicotine addiction, and in so doing, open a door to a higher level of awareness. The addiction effectively bypasses our rational thought processes by means of an interdependent structure of misperceptions that reinforce and compound each other. We inherit these slowly and imperceptibly, from a variety of sources. By correcting these erroneous patterns one becomes free from the addiction.

What I am not here to do is to reel off endless details of exactly how physically bad for you, nicotine is, or in what ways it damages the body.

The toxic properties of nicotine are both well documented and recognised, and it would be a waste for me to spend too much time reinforcing what everyone already knows. That said, I would be remiss if I didn't just give it a little space at this early stage of the journey.

Nicotine is:

"A very poisonous soluble fluid alkaloid with a pyridine-like odour and a burning taste, obtained from tobacco or produced synthetically. It is used as an agricultural insecticide, and in veterinary medicine as an external parasiticide"

(Dorland's illustrated Medical Dictionary)

Let's just stop for a moment and digest that. Nicotine, the drug that you are paying money to be addicted to, is quite literally also used to kill things. You spray it on insects, and they die. Outside its role in the tobacco and e-cigarette industries, nicotine is a chemical used directly for the purpose of inflicting death.

A dose of pure nicotine as low as 30mg can be fatal

And of course, let's not forget that in the case of tobacco, nicotine is by far not the only dangerous chemical that you are inhaling. Tobacco smoke is made up of thousands of chemicals, including at least 70 known to cause cancer. These include hydrogen cyanide, formaldehyde, lead, arsenic, ammonia, benzene and carbon monoxide. The list goes on:

"Cigarette smoking has been clearly and unambiguously identified as a direct cause of cancers of the oral cavity, oesophagus, stomach, pancreas, larynx, lung, bladder, kidney and leukaemia, especially acute myeloid leukaemia.'

Cigarette smoking is a direct cause of ischaemic heart disease (the commonest cause of death in western countries), respiratory heart disease, aortic aneurysm, chronic obstructive lung disease, stroke, pneumonia, and cirrhosis and cancer of the liver.

In developed countries as a whole, tobacco is responsible for 24% of all male deaths and 7% of all female deaths: these figures rise to over 40% in men in some countries of central and eastern Europe and to 17% in women in the United States. The average loss of life of smokers is 8 years. Tobacco is already the biggest cause of adult death in developed countries. Over the next few decades tobacco could well become the biggest cause of adult death in the world."

(Peter Boyle, Division of Epidemiology and Biostatistics, European Institute of Oncology, Milan, Italy)

I refer in this book primarily to smoking, but of course nicotine is also consumed via e-cigarettes ('vapes'), mouth sprays and nicotine patches, snüs and other methods. Generally speaking, official literature tends to classify people who smoke traditional cigarettes and people who vape, collectively as "smokers".

Nicotine is the common active ingredient across all of these delivery media. Whether cigarettes, vapes, or nicotine patches, the addiction is exactly the same, because the drug functions identically, however you consume it. If you have moved from cigarettes to vaping, you have obviously removed many of the harmful chemicals from the equation, but you are most certainly still in the grip of nicotine addiction. This book is also very much for you. Undoubtedly the absence of many of the toxic chemicals present in tobacco, does mean that vapes are physically less harmful than conventional cigarettes; however, nicotine is still the addictive component, and harmful in its own right. The active ingredient is the same, therefore the core concepts are identical. I am writing predominantly from the perspective of the smoker, because my personal experience of nicotine addiction is drawn from cigarettes. As it would feel clumsy to constantly say "smoking or vaping", or "tobacco or another nicotine delivery system" throughout the book you'll have to forgive me for sometimes simplifying things. My technique for breaking free of this addiction runs true across all methods of consuming nicotine. Vape or cigarette, patch or snü nicotine is the common denominator.

As you read the book you will come across examples which illustrate various aspects of nicotine addiction. It is very important that you scrutinise these examples meticulously. Even if they appear to be relatively simple, it is essential that you make an effort to clearly understand them and their implications.

The addiction is like a series of locks, which if unlocked correctly will open a door. If the keys are made properly, the door will open, and once opened it will remain that way. If, however, the keys are hastily or badly made, they may not work properly or even become jammed in the lock.

The examples I use are reflections of aspects of the addiction. By really making an effort to embrace them, the mechanics of the addiction will become clearer to you. If you simply scan something without properly absorbing it, you run the risk of failing to make crucial connections. This is not a book to be scanned. It is a book to read slowly and attentively, to fully understand what you are reading. This is the only way it will work.

When you read what seems to you to be a relatively simple situation, you might feel dismissive of it. You might feel that its simplicity means that it has no relevance to you and your complex addiction. This will be your ego taking control. Your ego is the area of your consciousness that deals with your sense of self-importance. It has a direct effect upon your perception of reality but should not be allowed to be the guiding factor in your decision-making process. Learning to recognise, observe and control your ego and its influence over you, is generally recognised as a fundamental aspect of spiritual practice. It is also a building block in the foundations of your freedom from nicotine addiction.

So try to apply a meticulous approach to your reading of the book as a whole. Do not be in a hurry. Take your time and read each sentence slowly and carefully, regularly asking yourself whether you have really understood. A lot of what you will read is deceptively simple and you may be tempted to move on without having grasped some vital subtlety. Observe your conscious reactions to what you are reading. Try to be objective about your responses. Step back and examine the thoughts that enter your mind. Ask yourself whether your responses are appropriate to what you are reading. You may read something and instinctively react in a specific way, but then on closer inspection discover that your reaction actually appears unnatural. You must make an effort to observe these reactions. To fully comprehend the mechanics of nicotine addiction, you must learn to gain a measure of control over your mind that has previously eluded you. You must learn to rise above your mind, step outside your emotions and observe yourself and your relationship to nicotine objectively. Imagine a model of a nicotine addict, something distinct from yourself. Try to observe that model, and how it behaves, with a degree of separation, if you can manage it.

Please note that I am not asking you to stop smoking or vaping while you are reading the book.

Within the realm of nicotine addiction, your ability to understand will be at its best when you are not influenced by cravings for the drug. Your transformation to the state of non-smoker will occur in its own time, irrespective of how much you smoke beforehand. It is better that you do not deny yourself until you find that it is no longer an issue of denial, but rather an emergence into a new state of consciousness, wherein smoking no longer plays a part. Just keep consuming nicotine until the addiction naturally ceases to function. Additionally, the observation and comprehension of the processes which constitute nicotine addiction, is the very essence of the method of freeing oneself from it, so actually smoking or vaping while reading the book, plays a part in that.

So above all, try to make your reading of this book an exercise in attentive reading. Read slowly and deliberately and make an extra effort to understand every nuance.

"If you wish to attain this true and genuine Way, you need to pay close attention to all the details."

Torei

In terms of an attitude with which to approach your reading, we might perhaps borrow a little from the Buddhist practice of Beginner's Mind. As the name suggests, this attitude encourages an abandoning of prior opinions, habitual reactions and judgements. This is a perfect attitude to adopt as one embarks on a voyage into liberation of the self from the bondage of addiction. Try to approach this process from a position of psychological and intellectual fertility around the subject. Empty, but with the potential to become newly full. Allow for the possibility that there is new information to absorb. No matter how much thought and effort you have given to this issue previously, allow for the possibility that there is something fundamental that you have missed. Allow for the possibility of a total sea-change in your foundational perception of smoking and nicotine addiction as a whole.

If you can understand what I have said in this chapter, then I promise you that you can become free from nicotine addiction forever. All you really require is comprehension.

If the basic language of this book is understandable to you, then liberation from nicotine is easily and permanently available as a direct result of what you will read here. The only thing that stands between you and freedom is your addicted mind.

The area of your consciousness that has become addicted to nicotine will resist the process. It will affect your concentration, blurring your focus as you read, attempting to distract you or to make you think that you have understood something when in fact you have not fully grasped it. On the basis of this, I advise a double-checking policy in your reading. Pause regularly and ask yourself whether you are fully in touch with what you have been shown. If you have not quite understood something, turn back and read again before proceeding. The truth is in here!

4

THE BREATH

The breath is the unifying factor common to both nicotine addiction and most, if not all, spiritual traditions. In Zen, awareness and counting of breath is a fundamental component of Zazen meditation. In the yogic traditions of India, the practice of pranayama is central, 'Prana' meaning Life Force, and 'Yama' meaning control. In Qigong, the breath is directed to and from the Dan Tien and other areas, to activate the Qi. In Mindfulness, meditation on breath is a foundational feature. The list goes on.

Given what we are dealing with here, then, it almost seems ridiculous to exclude some focus on our relationship to our breath, with regards the transcendence of nicotine addiction. After all, in almost all methods of consuming this drug, we are breathing it into our lungs. Given that the world's atmosphere is already heavily polluted, and that without oxygen we cannot stay alive, it seems the utmost folly to adulterate the air we are breathing further, with self-administered toxic chemicals. But if this wasn't a thing, I wouldn't be here writing this book. However, I think before we move further into this process, it would be good to take a few moments to remind ourselves exactly why it is that we are embarking on this journey. I invite you therefore to take a short time out from your reading, and sit with me in a simple meditation on the breath. If meditation isn't your thing, that's absolutely fine, you can skip past this. This isn't a part of the process, it's simply something that might help to foster a more receptive frame of mind as we begin the process.

Allow approximately 10 minutes, though feel free to take longer.

Choose a comfortable sitting position, wherever you are. It doesn't matter whether you are on a train, in the office, at home on a meditation cushion, or outside in a field; simply make yourself as comfortable as possible, preferably as upright as you can manage. You don't have to close your eyes, but I would recommend doing so, after you have read the next few paragraphs. If you don't want to, then at least lower and relax your gaze. Remember that in meditation we are paying attention, on purpose, in a particular kind of way, and trying to fall awake, rather than fall asleep. We are endeavouring to adopt an attitude of open acceptance and to be as non-judgemental as possible.

Start to notice your breathing. It's not something that we would ordinarily be aware of unless it is specifically drawn to our attention. Where is the sensation of breathing most noticeable to you? Is it around your nostrils and your mouth, where the air entering is cool, and warmer when leaving? Maybe it is in your chest, or lower down in your abdomen, where you might notice a gentle feeling of expansion as you breathe in, and contraction as you breathe out.

Once you have identified where you are most aware of your breathing, just allow your attention to remain there. Notice every in-breath, and every out-breath. Don't try to change the depth or pace of your breathing in any way. Just keep noticing it, in whatever way it happens.

It will of course be quite natural for your attention to wander as you are doing this, and you may find your awareness has shifted to something completely different. Don't worry at all about this. Simply acknowledge it, and gently lead yourself back to your breathing. It doesn't matter if your awareness wanders many times, just keep leading it back to your breath.

Allow your breathing awareness to continue for about ten minutes.

Then, before you open your eyes, just take a moment to consider exactly how precious your breath really is. Reflect on how something so gentle, so easy to forget about, is in fact what keeps you alive in this world. Place your hands on your chest or abdomen for a moment, and feel its rising and falling, and give thanks for your ability to breathe.

Hopefully wherever you were prior to this

meditation, you are now a little calmer, and in tune with your breath. Try to hold that awareness as you move forwards into this process. Consider your breath, clear and healthy, and how that is reflected in your whole nature. Think of it as a precious life-giving balm. The purer it is, the stronger your life-force. Reflect on the innate value of that. Consider, given how fundamental and how pure and specific the breath is, how contrary to the very nature of breathing it is to habitually adulterate it with a toxin.

I recommend, if you read this book in more than one sitting, come back to this meditation before each time you intend to start reading again. As the breath is the foundation of all meditation practice, so it should also be the foundation of your journey beyond this addiction, back to wholeness and health. Your breath is not meant to be held hostage to nicotine. Through the journey that lies ahead, we can liberate it once and for all.

5

Field of Vision

Imagine that you are looking at an image on a television screen. It shows some flowers. They are very pretty to look at, the whole image is beautiful. The flowers are a variety of colours, velvety petals shining in the sun. The camera filming the image is obviously in the air above the flowers, looking down upon them. The whole screen is filled with the image.

Now imagine that the camera filming the image pulls up from the flowers into the air, so that the image falls away, the flowers becoming smaller and smaller as the camera rises. As the camera moves higher, so the field of vision expands in every direction. As you look at the screen, you observe that the original patch of flowers is actually surrounded by many more flowers, in every direction. They were simply a small area of a large field of flowers. You observe that whilst the original patch of flowers was pretty to look at, the rest of the surrounding flowers in the field are in fact much prettier. The surrounding flowers are incredibly beautiful, beyond anything you have previously seen. Looking at the image of the field now, you can see that the original patch of flowers you were looking at is in fact a much less attractive area in the centre of a field of staggering beauty.

Viewed solely in their own context, the first image, the small patch of flowers, is a very pretty image. You can evaluate it in its own right, simply as a nice thing to look at, with no complications. Viewed in the context of the whole field, however, it is in fact the least attractive area of something much larger and more beautiful, yet in essence no more complicated.

Something quite simple can clearly be seen in radically different lights depending on whether we look at it in isolation or as part of a larger picture.

Imagine a beautiful, luxurious bed. If you lie in it, then physically you will immediately become comfortable. If, however, the bed is in a room, which you find particularly unpleasant, then your sense of comfort will be significantly undermined. It exists insofar as your body is in contact with something soft, but if you really can't stand the room then you will not experience much 'real' comfort at all. The aesthetic qualities of the room can influence how 'comfortable' you are as much as or even more than the more obvious physical softness of the bed. From this we can conclude that 'comfort' as a concept exists on two levels, the physical and the psychological.

This is the case with nicotine addiction. Just as your appreciation of the field of flowers, or the soft bed, depends on how much of the picture you can see, so your experience of smoking depends on how much genuine awareness you have of the underlying mechanism of nicotine addiction, beyond how it initially appears on the surface.

Many people try to give up without actually getting any better picture of what they are dealing with, without raising the camera. They don't realise that they can, and that it really changes things. Giving up smoking is not about effort, it is about awareness. It's not merely a matter of stopping lighting cigarettes and inhaling their smoke. Physically stopping yourself from smoking or vaping is not actually difficult, but if in actuality, you still want to do it and are missing the nicotine, then you haven't achieved very much in terms of how you feel. It is pointless *trying* to give up smoking, because a life of longing for something you cannot have is a life of torture, which nobody wants. All struggling should come to an end when you stop smoking. The real aim is to be free.

The appropriate emotional response to giving up smoking is one of joy and relief at having achieved something so positively transformative. Luckily this is attainable because if you stop correctly, by coming to understand with absolute clarity the nature of the conscious mechanism by which nicotine has wound itself into your life, then relief, release and happiness are inevitable. Think about it – you are not going to 'try' to give up smoking, miserably cutting down your intake day by day, longing and longing and gasping for a smoke. You can simply be free in an instant – exactly as long as it takes to understand something completely. Your understanding is the thing that has the power to set you free. If you really make a sincere effort to understand, then the end of your addiction is only as far away as a bit of clear and honest thinking.

It is not enough simply to arrive at a point of confidence and think "excellent, now I am sure that I will be able to give up smoking" That might on the face of things appear to be a very constructive state of mind, but what you are aiming for is correct and total understanding, because only then does an instantaneous transformation take place. Total understanding can take you directly to the position of the non-smoker, by-passing all that tedious 'trying to give up' with its withdrawal pangs and stress and so on. One minute you are a smoker; the next minute you were a smoker. So quick you almost missed it, but there it was, that tiny momentary spark of absolute realization that is worth a lifetime of being 'pretty much sure', of something.

By approaching it in the right way – and I'm going to take you there in this book – the transition from the state of the nicotine addict to that of permanent non-smoker should be as straightforward as the flicking of a switch. In reality there are only two states: smoker and non-smoker. It is not really relevant whether you vape or smoke once a year or once a minute, the issue is your conceptual perception of consuming nicotine as a whole. If you can accept the idea of consuming it in any way at all, then you are in the conscious condition of the nicotine addict. You are accepting smoking as valid in some way, and the fundamental position of the non-smoker is that of absolute rejection of smoking. It requires no effort whatsoever, as it is an instinctive response, as natural as breathing, and sits at the foundational level of our perception of reality.

The states of smoker and non-smoker are both simply the product of our level of understanding of tobacco and/or nicotine, and since one can come to understand something in an instant, one may also become an ex-nicotine addict in the same amount of time

It is easy to underestimate the power that lies in truth.

Realising the truth about nicotine addiction is the key to becoming free of it. From the moment you first glimpse the truth, you have set something in motion in yourself, which will not be held back. It is like a fuse which once lit will inevitably burn to its end. You determine the length of the fuse. You can choose to bring things to an end simply by thinking clearly and honestly. When you wholeheartedly embrace the truth, you will be a non-smoker.

We are not dealing with belief here - 'believing' you can achieve something. We are dealing with knowledge – solid, absolute awareness, which simply is, and as such occupies its correct place among the foundations of your life. Your understanding and whole view of nicotine in any form will come to sit permanently alongside such basic concepts as: "Gravity pulls me forcefully towards the centre of the Earth, therefore I avoid falling from great heights." or "I do not pick up shit from the ground and eat it because it will make me ill.", and so on. It is that simple. No stress, no withdrawal symptoms, just "Wow! I don't smoke anymore. That's all there is to it after all that fuss. So simple, it was right under my nose the whole time. I actually have done it! No more of this endless thinking about giving up smoking; I now actually am a non- smoker! Now I can finally get excited about what it is going to feel like never to smoke again!"

Let me illustrate exactly how easy it is going to be. Imagine that every morning somebody brings you a nice cup of tea in bed (or coffee, juice, Martini, whatever). You love your morning cup of tea, and look forward to it eagerly. It is your reassuring start to the day. Then I say to you "OK, now I want you to say 'No' to that cup of tea every morning from now on". The person is still going to carry on bringing the tea to you and offering it to you, but from now on, every time they do, you must decline and go without. Now obviously you could do this. To say 'No' to a cup of tea every morning is not beyond your capabilities. But if you wanted that cup of tea, then it would be a pretty miserable, frustrating state of affairs. It would make you unhappy but you could do it. This is what is happening when you are 'trying to give up smoking'. You can do it, but it does not make you happy.

Nothing has really been achieved in terms of establishing a long-lasting positive state of mind, and it's that positive state of mind that pays the biggest dividend in actual health and well-being.

If, however, I were to inform you that the person who brings you the cup of tea actually spits in the cup before they enter the room, then things would be different. If I also provided you with all the necessary apparatus to make your own drink, from the comfort of your bed, thus enabling you to gain control of the situation for yourself, would you then still accept the offered tea that has been spat in?

Saliva-fetishists aside, you would not. Would you be missing out on anything? No, you would miss nothing at all. You would still have your tea every morning exactly as you like it, but through the correct information, you are able to make a rational choice and say 'No' to the cup of tea which has been spat in. That same, original, adulterated tea will still be offered to you every morning, but now you are more aware of the whole of the situation.

Admittedly things look the same, but you now know that they aren't. There is no way that, once you have been made aware of the fact that the person is spitting in your tea, you are going to somehow forget and accidentally drink the tea with the spit in it!! How could you? It is such a fundamental fact that you couldn't forget. Once you become aware, your understanding of the situation is permanently changed.

This is knowledge of a situation. You know now that the person spits in the tea before they give it to you. Additionally, you also have a perfectly good cup of tea, which you have made yourself. It is now very easy to say no to the cup of tea that you are offered every morning, though nothing has changed about the way in which you are offered the tea, or its appearance.

Only your perception of the event has changed, in the light of new information.

This change of perception is the key to the situation, and in exactly the same way, a change of perception is the key to conquering nicotine addiction. Take some time to consider and re-read carefully this situation that I have just described, and make absolutely sure that you clearly understand it. It is easy to read something straightforward and not absorb it fully. Think about your view of the situation before and after I told you that the person was spitting in the tea, and how differently the situation looks, before and after becoming aware of this. On the surface, it all appears the same, but the level of change is actually profound. You will have lost nothing and gained what you always really wanted from the situation.

If I had initially asked you "Could you say no to this cup of tea every morning?" before you were aware of all the facts, then you would probably have replied "Yes, I could say no, but I would regret it because I would want the tea". If I asked you after I had informed you of the facts and equipped you with your own tea-making facilities, then your reply would probably be something more like "Of course I could refuse the tea. Why would I possibly think of saying yes, when not only am I aware that it has been spat in, I am also in possession of a perfectly good cup of tea which contains all of the positive factors of the original cup, but without any saliva in it!"

This situation is a model for the way in which you will come to understand and overcome nicotine addiction. When you think about giving up smoking without adequate information, you see it in much the same way as that initial cup of tea, but when the real facts of the situation come to light, it changes in the same way. You will suddenly come to realise that you have thought that something was one way, whereas actually it is another, and this simple understanding will make smoking utterly irrelevant to you. In addition, you will also see that the thing you thought you stood to lose by stopping smoking, will not be lost; it will actually be gained in a more complete form. It will not be a matter of 'trying to stop smoking', because you will not see smoking in the same way at all.

6

THE 'SELF DESTRUCTIVE STREAK'

In a sense, there is only one conversation which can be had about smoking, since there is simply one set of facts that make up the issue. Obviously, you can vary the order in which you address the various aspects, but fundamentally it is a pretty cut-and-dried matter. The conversation, if seen through to its conclusion, must inevitably end with the person who is a smoker becoming a non-smoker. This is because smoking and the understanding of the nature of smoking are mutually incompatible. It is not possible to smoke if you understand smoking any more than it is possible to point a loaded gun at your face and pull the trigger if you know what guns do.

"Ah yes, but that's what I like, it's that self-destructive streak in me that makes me smoke."

This is a very common assumption that people make about their motivation to smoke, but it doesn't really stand up.

In most cases, we start to smoke or vape because we think that we are going to experience something positive. We do not generally choose to do things on the basis that they do us harm. If you started smoking because you thought it might be nice, then to turn round later and claim that you smoke out of some kind of self-loathing makes no sense. It is nicotine addiction, which affects the way we think, which leads us to believe that we are acting out of some kind of desire for self-harm. We start out as innocent pleasure-seekers, but as nicotine eats away our vitality, we acquire a more morbid attitude. We are moving closer to death, so we become more deathly in our nature. We spend the whole of our time harming ourselves for the sake of benefits that are wholly illusory. Our misinformed condition means that we are driven to validate our relationship with smoking for the sake of our own self-esteem, so we construct reasons to excuse ourselves, which are born out of the things we are actually doing. We are effectively inflicting a fair measure of harm on ourselves with absolutely no gain whatsoever. In terms of our actions, we are a self-destructive person. In terms of our real selves, though, we are still the innocent individuals who took that first cigarette in the search for a new uplifting experience with which to enrich our lives.

To blame smoking on a self-destructive trait in your personality is weak thinking.

"Ah well, that's just me, I'm just too weak then, so I guess I'll just have to carry on smoking."

You are not weak, you are inherently strong, but nicotine addiction is something that affects the whole of your consciousness, so that you actually appear, to yourself, to agree with ludicrously insupportable arguments for carrying on smoking! Your mental and emotional faculties are fundamentally compromised by the addiction. Smoking makes you weaker, so you come to think of yourself as inherently weak, because you can't stop doing the thing that is harming you. The reason you cannot stop, though, is nothing to do with strength, or weakness, it is an issue of comprehension.

The nature of nicotine is not readily explained to us. The risks from smoking are well publicised, but they mean little, because we are accustomed to making a sacrifice in order to gain something, so smoking seems little different from most things we choose to do or not to do.

To make someone aware only of the risks from doing something can be a smokescreen to avoid focusing on the certainties. If someone offers you the chance to do something which may be harmful, then you will be more likely to accept the offer if the person making it admits that there are risks involved. They appear to have given you information that would not normally incline you towards their offer. You feel confident in accepting what the person is offering because their surrender to you of negative information gives you the feeling that you are in possession of the facts of the situation. You are told 'this may happen', or 'that may happen', but always the inference is there that these negative factors should be acceptable to us because of what we get out of these other positive things that will also happen. The positive things themselves, however, are never openly promoted in anything other than a largely abstract way. The tobacco and e-cigarette industries argue that people have freedom of choice to smoke or not to smoke. Freedom of choice, however, is dependent on being fully aware of the implications of the choices one is considering. Freedom of choice is making a decision based on an appreciation of the facts. Because some negative facts about nicotine/tobacco are made publicly available, we tend to assume that we have been made aware of the whole truth. In this frame of mind, we start to smoke, feeling that the responsibility for this course of action lies solely with ourselves.

It is unwise to assume that simply because one has been made aware of information about something, one is aware of the whole situation.

A Zen student came to Bankei and complained: "Master, I have an ungovernable temper. How can I cure it?"

"You have something very strange," replied Bankei. "Let me see what you have."

"Just now I cannot show it to you," replied the other.

"When can you show it to me?" asked Bankei.

"It arises unexpectedly," replied the student.

"Then," concluded Bankei, "it must not be your own true nature. If it were, you could show it to me at any time. When you were born you did not have it, and your parents did not give it to you. Think that over."

7

WHY DO WE ENJOY SMOKING?

People often comment that they would like to give up smoking but they enjoy it too much, or that they don't want to stop because they enjoy it so much. I am not denying that it can be pleasurable, but there is more to understand than is at first apparent. We need to examine first why it is that we enjoy it so much and what is the nature of the enjoyment.

Essentially it is that lift, that sensation of being more relaxed, more focussed, less angry, more able to deal with whatever you are currently seeking to deal with. It can very much be said to be directly 'performance-related', in that whenever you arrive at a situation in which you need to be operating efficiently as a person, your system automatically craves nicotine in response to the system's demands. You smoke a cigarette, and sure enough you feel better - more able to focus on the situation in hand.

When I talk about 'operating more efficiently as a person', I am speaking in a very broad sense. For instance, one might equally need to perform efficiently in order to relax well as much as one might need to in order to perform a complicated task well.

This of course seems like a pretty reasonable

argument for smoking. Something that simply makes you feel and perform better than you do normally, must be a good thing.

Obviously, if this were what actually occurred, then it would be excellent. You might well justifiably accept many negative effects for the sake of the obvious benefits. The real situation, however, is a little more complex. We have to take a step back from the basic act of smoking a cigarette and what that does for you on an immediate level, and understand the bigger picture, in much the same way as to wholly appreciate the flowers I mentioned, we must view them in the context of the whole field.

Nicotine is an incredibly subtle drug. It is both highly addictive and yet very simple to give up when approached correctly. The addiction has two aspects, the physical and the psychological. The two are obviously fundamentally linked. Essentially, the physical side of the addiction tends to activate in response to the triggers of mental-emotional responses to given situations. For instance, you enter a situation of stress. Your subconscious mind immediately makes an association - "stress - I need some nicotine". This triggers your physical addiction and you begin to physically desire the satisfying bodily sensation that the cigarette will give you. Mentally, you immediately respond, thinking "Yes, smoke a cigarette now and I will become less stressed and feel much better in general." You smoke a cigarette. Sure enough, you experience an immediate lessening in your stress levels and are thus able to deal more efficiently with the stress-situation in which you have found yourself. Physically you feel more balanced and at ease.

So, it seems that as a smoker, you basically feel pretty much normal most of the time, but when you need a little lift, tobacco gives you that extra support that you need to get you through.

An appealing scenario, but this is not actually what is happening.

Imagine a person who buys a house and is very happy with it and thinks, "This is a very good thing which has happened to me". They have a nice house. This is good. However, if the land on which the house is built then subsides and the house collapses, then the person has lost everything. Although at the time the person was happy with the purchase of the house and thought it a very good thing, viewed retrospectively, it was a very bad thing to have happened.

Similarly, imagine a person who is left by their partner whom they love passionately. The relationship is over. The person who has been rejected is very sad and thinks, "This is a very bad thing which has happened to me". Relative to this moment in their life and judged only in the terms of his or her perception that they wanted this relationship to continue, a bad thing has indeed happened to this person. They no longer have the relationship they wanted, and they are heartbroken. However, imagine this person is a songwriter and the depth of the emotions triggered by the break-up cause them to write a song so heartfelt that it becomes a hit-selling record. Later they meet someone else and fall in love again and realize that they have found a much more fulfilling relationship than the previous one. They are now even happier than they were in the old relationship. Now, when we look at the original break-up and ask, "Was that a bad thing to have happened or a good thing?" we can see that although it seemed bad at the time, it was in fact a very good thing, which took place.

So it is with smoking. Even though it appears to be helping at the time, the reality is that on a greater scale, something far more sinister is occurring, which when grasped wholeheartedly, makes the immediate benefits every bit as deceptive as the initial events in both of the above examples.

A common factor amongst addictive drugs is the way in which the user, after a time, comes to need the drug simply to feel normal, rather than deriving any pleasure from it. This is not exactly a universal rule, but a theme that appears to some extent across the spectrum of addictive substances. The differences vary from drug to drug. There are usually differences in time-scale. For instance, a heroin user may experience this over a period of weeks or months, whilst a cocaine user might find after only a few hours they are taking the drug simply to prolong a state of normality, rather than intoxication, this being preferable than confronting the unpleasant period of withdrawal. Even with alcohol, we talk sometimes of people "drinking themselves sober". Nicotine is an interesting combination of factors, in that it appears to become more enjoyable over time, whilst actually it is following much the same pattern as other addictive drugs.

Take a look at the next illustration, (fig.1 page 42)

The horizontal axis of the graph is simply your movement forwards through life. The vertical axis is a measure of how 'whole' you are feeling at any given time. I mean this in both a physical and psychological sense – an overall sense of well-being. Obviously, the higher up the vertical axis, the better you are feeling – the more 'in the light.'

As you can see, there are two paths shown on the picture. The person on the lower path is a smoker. You can see that the path of the smoker is gradually heading downhill into darkness. The constant ingestion of nicotine into their bloodstream is making them feel gradually less whole, as they become less healthy. You can also see that when the person on the lower path smokes a cigarette, their path briefly turns uphill. They feel better for a short while, but then they once more head downhill again into the darkness. From this we can observe that the smoker does feel more together when they smoke a cigarette.

If we look at the higher path, that of the non-smoker, we can see that they are not heading

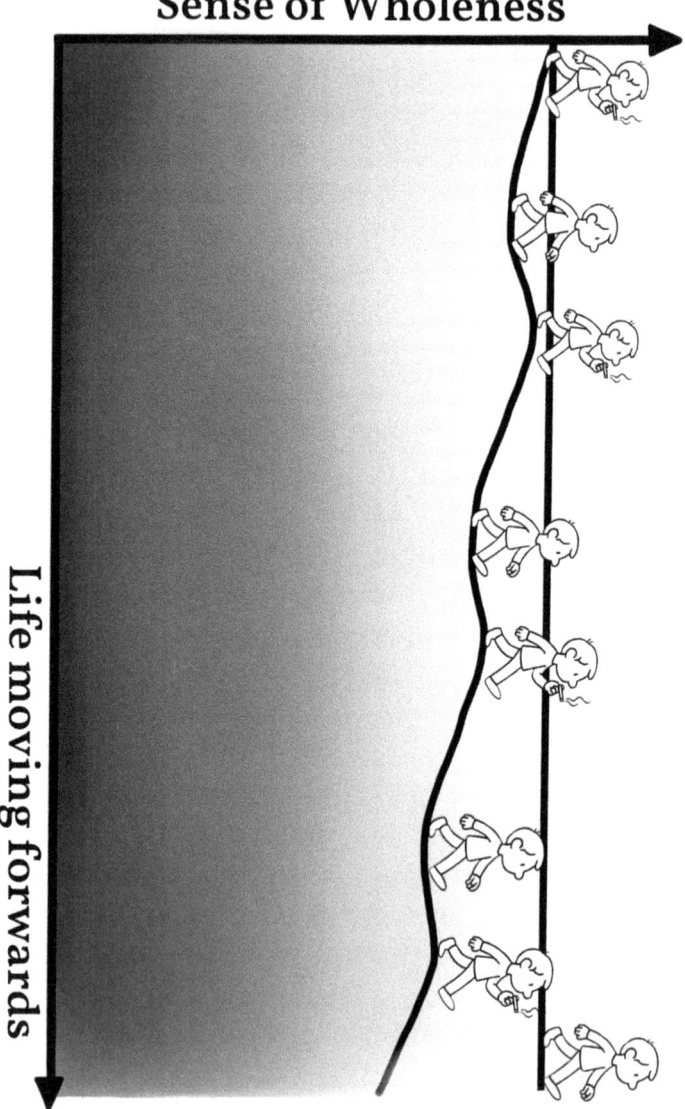

Fig 1

downhill in the same way. The non-smoker is not drip-feeding toxic chemicals into their bloodstream, and therefore they walk an even path, forwards, in clarity. Smoking is not dragging them slowly downhill into darkness.

Looking at the two paths in relation to each other, the point is simple. Smokers and non-smokers begin at the same level. The smokers, however, are gradually heading down into a darker state of lesser clarity. They gradually feel less whole. Although smoking a cigarette does make them feel better at the time, it is still only taking them up towards the level at which the non-smoker exists constantly. The improvement in how whole the smoker feels is only an improvement in relation to the point at which the cigarette is smoked. The path turns uphill, but only because the nicotine has taken it downhill in the first place. Relative to the normal state of a non-smoker, they still feel worse generally. From the point of view of the smoker, however, the rate of descent is so slow as to be imperceptible from day to day, so that the illusion of normality interspersed with uplifting cigarettes, is a convincing one.

So why then do we enjoy smoking so much, and what is the nature of that enjoyment?

We enjoy smoking so much because we enjoy being alive. The enjoyment is completely natural, because it is natural to enjoy a return to a more normal state of being. If you have the flu and then become well again, you enjoy the sensation of becoming well again. If you are dependent on nicotine and fulfil that need, then you enjoy the fulfilment. The illusion lies in our perception that we were already feeling normal before smoking the cigarette and that it has made us feel better than normal. The reality is that we were not feeling normal before smoking the cigarette and that by smoking it we have moved closer to a state of normality. This is bound to be enjoyable. It is enjoyable to be more focused. It is enjoyable to feel less stressed. The nature of the enjoyment we derive from consuming nicotine is that it is the sensation of a return to a normal state of being which has been lost through the consumption of nicotine in the first place.

The fact is that the sensation that you experience when you smoke a cigarette is effectively a small glimpse of what it feels like to be a non-smoker, since a non-smoker feels normal all of the time rather than simply after they have smoked. The driving desire that lies at the heart of nicotine addiction is for the feeling that ironically can only be fully attained by not being a nicotine addict.

8

STRESS

Perhaps the most common reason that we give for smoking is that it helps to relieve stress.

If you are addicted to nicotine, then when you enter a situation that causes you stress, smoking a cigarette will on an immediate level make you less stressed. But, nicotine itself actually undermines the nervous system, by virtue of its inherent toxicity. This therefore not only induces stress, but also renders you very gradually less capable of dealing with anything, as the volume-control on your vitality is turned ever downwards. By smoking the cigarette, or inhaling the vape, the immediate stress has been reduced but the net effect of doing this is that the damage done to the nervous system by ingesting the dose of nicotine will actually induce more stress in the long run than the cigarette has alleviated. If you smoke then you can expect the amount of stress in your life to be far greater, even though smoking appears to be easing it.

The thing that you believe to be the cure, is actually the cause.

This is why cigarette smoking accelerates over time, because obviously the system gradually becomes less and less healthy, so stress levels tend to be higher, so more pangs for smoking are triggered, so more cigarettes/vapes are smoked, so more stress is induced and so on and on and on. Thus of course we can see how the classic image of the super-stressed, high-speed chain smoker comes about: it is the obvious conclusion – a person totally locked into smoking, finding reasons for stress in everything around them, but never realising that the stress is the ironic product of the thing they cling to - the one little prop they see as their lifeline in this ocean of stress!

"But how do you know that nicotine causes stress? What are you, some kind of medical expert?"

You don't need to be a medical expert to understand that ingesting nicotine causes stress, any more than you need to be a mechanic to understand that a car won't run properly if you put dishwater in the petrol tank. It's too simple to require expertise. Wherever you sit in terms of the location of the self (that's another story), I'm sure we can all agree that the human brain plays a fundamental part in processing our thoughts and feelings. Perhaps it might be said to mediate between the self, the mind and the outside world. The brain is an organ in the body, and like all organs, it requires blood to function. If the blood you feed your brain is constantly adulterated with a toxic chemical (or in the case of tobacco, multiple toxic chemicals), it will inevitably become gradually less healthy. Its functioning will be sub-optimal, with a progressive decline. Ergo it follows that whatever we ask of the brain under these conditions, it will be less able to achieve. There is no way that constantly drip-feeding toxin into your brain, is going to lead to an increase in positivity. Quite the opposite. The decline in health of the brain, will inevitably entail a commensurate decline in emotional state to match – an increase in stress, anxiety, paranoia; any and all negative emotional states - as the brain becomes gradually less able to function properly.

Fig.2 illustrates the cyclic relationship of nicotine and stress:

Nicotine Addiction in Motion

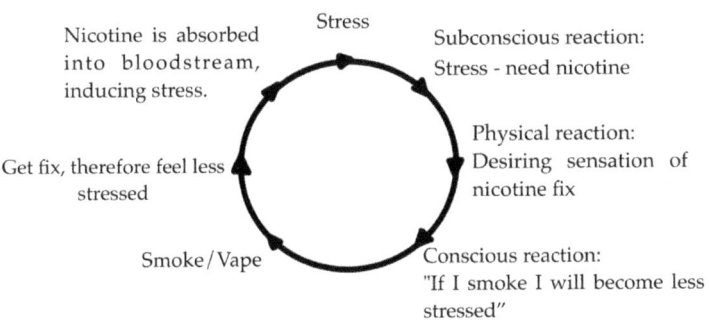

Nicotine is absorbed into bloodstream, inducing stress.

Stress

Subconscious reaction: Stress - need nicotine

Physical reaction: Desiring sensation of nicotine fix

Get fix, therefore feel less stressed

Smoke / Vape

Conscious reaction: "If I smoke I will become less stressed"

Fig 2

Stress is also a major difficulty for people trying to give up smoking without complete information.

In fig.3, you can see how stress snowballs when we try to stop by willpower alone. The stress from stopping smoking is mostly caused by misinformation about smoking itself. If you do not fully understand what you are dealing with, then you make the wrong associations. The reason that people find it stressful trying to stop smoking is that they are mistaken about what smoking/vaping actually does, and so they feel they no longer have something they need. The sense of loss caused by this erroneous mind-set causes the person to experience stress. Since they associate tobacco directly with relief of stress, denying themselves the thing that they think they need to ease their stress induces more stress, to which they react in

Trying To Give Up By Willpower Alone

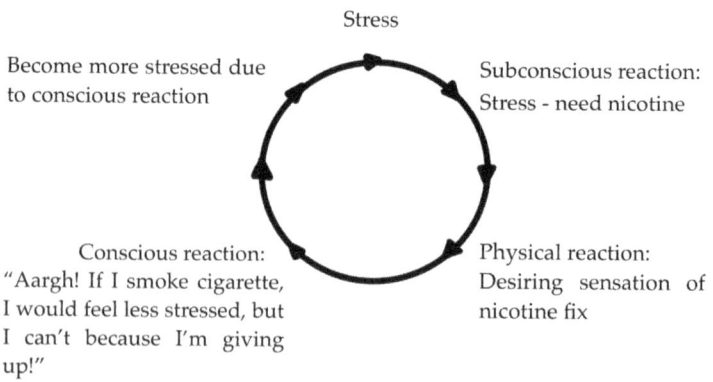

Fig 3

Giving Up Smoking With Understanding

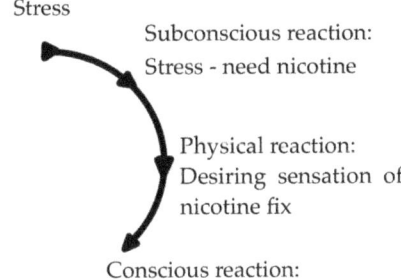

Stress

Subconscious reaction:
Stress - need nicotine

Physical reaction:
Desiring sensation of
nicotine fix

Conscious reaction:

If I feel as though if I smoke/vape, I will feel less stressed, and if I smoke now, I will appease my addiction, so I will feel less stressed.

In the long run, however, that will actually make me more stressed since I will have ingested a dose of nicotine, which actually causes stress.

If I don't smoke, however, I won't ingest any more nicotine, and will therefore take myself genuinely nearer to the state that I am mistakenly looking to the cigarette/vape to provide me with. By not smoking I will permanently reduce my stress levels. I can overcome my subconscious urge to smoke by rationalising it in this way and become calmer as I know that I am finally overcoming my addiction and never be stressed in this way again.

Fig 4

much the same way. The result is that the stress snowballs, feeding itself.

The fact is that smoking does not cure stress; it induces it. It only appears to cure stress, because once you are addicted to it, you need it to be able to operate more efficiently (feel normal), so when you smoke in a stress situation, you receive a dose of nicotine, move nearer to your optimum state and therefore resultantly become less stressed. 'Less stressed' is the natural human condition which nicotine takes away from you by enslaving and destroying your nervous system.

It is a self-reinforcing chain of illusion, which simply runs on and on until it is broken by understanding.

9

'Giving Up'

"I gave up once, and yes I did feel better, but in the end, I decided I still preferred what smoking does for me, so I started again."

Let's face it, you never 'gave up', because if you had actually 'given up', then by definition you would not have started again. To 'give up' means 'to stop', not 'to stop and then start again after a while!' In this case it would be more accurate to say "I paused smoking for a while".

The state of the 'non-smoker' is largely psychological. It is dependent on actually being fully conscious of the fact that not only do you not smoke, but that you never will smoke and in fact could never smoke.

It is the delusional blindness of the addiction itself within us, and its stranglehold on our ego, that tries to suppose that by merely stopping smoking for a while, we have overcome nicotine addiction. The state of non-smoker, in a permanent sense, is the inevitable result of understanding nicotine addiction. To assume that because you have physically stopped inhaling cigarettes or vapes, you must have totally understood nicotine addiction is to take a purely mechanistic view of the situation. If the only measure of the control over you that the addiction has were whether or not you are performing the physical act of smoking or vaping, then you would be correct, but the physical aspect of the addiction is really just an outward expression of the psychological aspect.

It is totally possible to stop smoking for the rest of your life, but to remain a nicotine addict to the grave.

The addiction takes control of your ego, and your ego will take affront at the 'outrageous' suggestion that you, who stopped smoking once for one whole year could possibly have anything more to learn about smoking! However, if there is any way that you can possibly consider smoking as something you have some chance of doing again, if you feel any pull of desire towards tobacco, or nicotine in any form at all, then there is something more for you to learn.

Really there is everything more to learn, because nicotine addiction is in essence a psychological issue and as such cannot be overcome by purely physical means. There are only two states – smoker and non-smoker. You are either one or the other. The transition from one to the other is instantaneous. You can catch momentary glimpses of the truth in advance of its full realization, but for everyone there comes a single moment of absolute clarity, when you truly understand, and there is no going back from that moment.

10

GRADUAL CHANGE

One of the reasons it is hard to discern exactly what it is that smoking is doing to us is that the change is a very gradual one. As smokers, we do basically feel largely OK for most of the time, and when we actually smoke a cigarette, it does make us feel better, so the daily reality is not difficult to deal with and it is easy to invest faith in this state of affairs. The fall down from 100% is not a sharp drop - this is the way the deception works. We only very gradually become less healthy. The decline is so gradual that we accept the way we are feeling as normality, because the rate of change is too slow for us to really register it. Consider the movement of the hour hand of a clock. It is imperceptibly slow, but although our senses are not equipped to register such a pace, we do not deny that it moves round the clock face twice a day. It is surprising how easily we can forget the way we felt in the distant past, so it is easy to convince ourselves that nothing has changed. Think about it though. On a basic level, for as long as you are a smoker, you are not simply a person. You are a person whose body has had their bloodstream diluted with toxic chemicals over a long period of time. The blood, which feeds your brain, is not simply blood; it is a mixture of blood and carcinogenic poison. Your essence has been adulterated. This drug is so subtle and sinister that whilst all it actually does is to make you feel a little worse than you should, it creates the illusion that it is making you feel better, because you are in such a state of symbiosis with it that you need it to feel normal! This is not in any way a normal condition to be in. To assume that you ever feel anywhere near your optimum state in this condition is ridiculous. You exist in a sub-optimal state, punctuated by momentary glimpses of how you are supposed to feel. You just didn't notice the decline, because it was stretched out over a really long period of time, normality slipping away from you in tiny increments, the rate of change too slow for human perception to register.

11

For/Against

Let us look at smoking/vaping in terms of reasons for and against:

AGAINST:
A significant chance of dying from it.
Costs lots of money.
Prevents you from experiencing what it feels like to be a normal healthy person.
Doesn't actually do anything anyway, apart from make you feel worse than you are supposed to.

FOR:
Helps you to relax, relieves stress, makes you more together etc.
Gives you something to do with your hands.
Tastes nice.
Helps you to fit in/be different.

So, against, we have the obvious significant chance of dying from it. This is probably greater in the case of smoking over vaping, but nonetheless either way one consumes a toxic drug, and in the case of vaping, the jury is still out as to the long-term effects, but it isn't looking good on current evidence. So as well as the ill-health which occurs whether or not you actually die; the fact that it costs you lots of money, perhaps most importantly the fact that it prevents you from experiencing the simple sensation of being a normal healthy human being, and of course the ridiculous fact that for all its great claims, it doesn't actually do anything (apart from making you feel slightly worse than you would otherwise feel).

So what does the 'For' side have to say for itself?

IT HELPS YOU TO RELAX, RELIEVES STRESS, MAKES YOU FEEL MORE TOGETHER, AND SO ON.

Except that it doesn't.

It only appears to do that because it creates the illusion that it is making you feel better by first making you feel worse than you should whilst simultaneously developing a dependency upon it which results in your needing it to feel anywhere near normal!

IT GIVES YOU SOMETHING TO DO WITH YOUR HANDS.

Let's all risk a significant chance of death, spend loads of money, and spend the whole of our lives feeling less happy or healthy than we are supposed to, so that we can have something to do with our hands! I don't think so. The opposite is in fact true. Far from giving us something to do with our hands, cigarettes tend to stop us from being able to do anything with our hands, even relax them. They just get in the way, so if we want to do anything with our hands, we have to find somewhere to put the cigarette.

IT TASTES NICE.

Except it doesn't.

Let's deal with this one right now. We must remember that all of the supposed benefits of cigarettes are purely relative to the world of the nicotine addict. Try to remember the very first time you ever really inhaled tobacco. Did it taste nice?

Of course not, you coughed your lungs out and your eyes watered and you felt terrible, and all your friends laughed and told you reassuringly – "It's all right, you just have to get into it!"

I can remember my first cigarette very clearly. I lived in the countryside at the time, and we were hiding out in the fields behind a wall. My friend had managed to steal a couple of his Mum's cigarettes and we had sneaked off to try them. I remember feeling very excited. Cigarettes seemed very rebellious, like some kind of forbidden fruit; so stepping over the line into the world of smoking seemed very attractive.

I remember specifically my first 'drag' on the cigarette. I instantly managed to inhale the smoke, having watched enough adults do it to get an idea of what you were supposed to do. I sucked the smoke into my lungs. I felt as though something had exploded inside my chest, the explosion spreading quickly to my head. I coughed violently and simultaneously thought:

That tastes terrible

What was all the fuss about?

Hooray, now I smoke and I feel very cool and rebellious.

So there we are. It tasted terrible, but I was already so psychologically worked up about the whole concept that I was still able to feel good about it. All I thought was "Ah well, it tastes horrible, but everyone says that after a while you get into it, so I guess if I stick with it then things will improve!" **There's the key phrase: "You have to get into it."**

So, something which at first experience tastes horrible, makes you cough painfully and which in fact your body totally rejects, you have to 'get into'. What does this mean? If you keep at it, it will change and you will come to like it? How so? How is this possible? Over a period of time, as you become a more 'expert' smoker, you will learn to alter the chemical content of tobacco so that it changes from something which simply tastes terrible to something which makes you feel good and tastes OK? Sounds ridiculous, but if one 'gets into' smoking, then presumably something of this sort must be happening.

What actually happens is that you try it, it is terrible, but because psychologically you are already hooked, you keep on doing it until you have hammered your system into a state of dependency upon it, so that then you come to need it, therefore it starts to taste and make you feel good. When you get it, you are satisfying your desire. Once you are dependent, the smoke entering your mouth and lungs, is accompanied by a rush as your craving is fulfilled and you move back towards your optimum capacity. It tastes good in much the same way that life tastes good, because 'life' is the commodity that nicotine is stealing from you and then selling back to you in far lesser quantities than you need at a greater price than you can afford.

Now obviously this picture is a little more nuanced in the case of vapes over cigarettes. With vapes, the nicotine has been separated from the accompanying baggage of the rest of the constituents of tobacco, and the additional chemicals added to cigarettes, and is hidden behind a screen of flavouring. But nonetheless, people starting vaping also most often cough a lot at the start, before gradually adjusting to the experience, at which point the cough recedes. This is especially the case if they are approaching nicotine for the first time in this way, as opposed to migrating from tobacco.

This change really does occur, but it cannot be because tobacco or vapes change, and if something is fundamentally bad and then starts to seem good, then to simply assume that you have 'got into' the thing is a very naive interpretation of the situation. We cannot suppose that we have become 'better' at smoking/vaping and have somehow 'learnt' to take advantage of nicotine's hidden property to make us feel better.

Think about it.

Think about my first smoking experience that I

described. Under normal circumstances, a person experimenting with something new is a pretty straightforward matter. In most cases if you try something and find it unpleasant, then you do not carry on doing it, unless there is some obvious reason to persevere, such as at a gymnasium in order to become fit. I, however, tried something, found it unpleasant, but resigned myself to carrying on doing it, reassuring myself that with time it would improve! It did not occur to me simply to not do it again because it wasn't very nice. It gave me no sensory fulfilment whatsoever, but psychologically I was addicted before I had even lit a cigarette. When I finally smoked, it was enough that I had done something that I had been conditioned to feel I should do, to assure me that I would carry on smoking. I actually convinced myself that it was a positive experience. It made my head spin, due to the brief increase in my heart rate and blood pressure, and it made me feel 'cool' due to the brief appeasement of my ego. I was already psychologically addicted to nicotine before I had ever smoked.

This is a very real aspect of the overall situation. It is perfectly possible for someone to effectively spend their entire life as a nicotine addict, whilst never actually smoking a cigarette. I have observed this situation in action occasionally, when I have wound up in conversation with someone who actively argues pro-smoking issues without ever actually having smoked. You do not have to do something to be under illusions as to the nature of that thing. It is perfectly possible to refrain from doing something but always to harbour some desire to do it, based on your observations of other people doing it. Obviously somebody in this situation is not suffering the health risks that a smoker is, but they are still in a state of illusion about something really important. They are part of a self-reinforcing web of misinformation, which enshrouds the world.

If you want to test this matter of whether or not cigarettes actually taste good then try the following:

Wait until you want a cigarette. Light and smoke one. As soon as you have finished smoking it, light and smoke another one. Smoke all of it. As soon as you have finished this one, light and smoke another one. Repeat until sick. This exercise obviously can be replicated with a vape. It might take a bit longer to arrive at the conclusion, but the pattern is identical.

The first one of course does make you feel better. You wanted one. Your system, which depends on them to feel normal, craved one. You smoked one, so your addiction was fulfilled. Your system was consequently able to operate more effectively and thus you felt more 'normal', i.e. better than you did before smoking the cigarette.

The second cigarette probably doesn't taste as good as the first; and the third, well let's face it, it really tastes pretty awful.

What has changed?

The cigarettes were identical, but each one had a progressively worse effect on you. How is this? If we examine the situation from the point of view that the cigarette itself does make you feel better, then this progressive decline in pleasure in the ones you have just smoked is a little hard to explain.

It really is simple though. Initially your addicted system needs a dose of nicotine to feel more normal. You smoke, receive your dose, and consequently you feel closer to how you are meant to feel i.e. better than you did before smoking the cigarette. Obviously people and their levels of addiction differ, but at some point, your craving for nicotine is fully appeased; whether it is by the end of the first cigarette/vape, or the third, or the tenth. The point is that if you keep smoking them immediately one after the other, you will inevitably reach saturation point. In terms of the graph, you have already reached the top of the peak (see fig 1 on page 42), so with subsequent doses of nicotine you have no further to go. You have already returned as near as you can get to normality and therefore, because nicotine is not actually something which improves your condition in any way, the subsequent cigarettes or vapes are illustrating for you the actual effect of smoking – it makes you feel bad. It tastes bad – end of story.

So, back to our FOR/AGAINST list. All we have left to look at on the 'FOR' side is that it helps you to fit in/be different – the social aspect of the drug.

As participants in modern, ego-driven society, we tend towards slavery to our self-image. Appearances are everything, and that begins with how we view ourselves. We all in a sense seek to be the God of our own personal universe. We seek acceptance from our peers; but at the same time we want to define ourselves as independent individuals. Smoking and vaping have cleverly manoeuvred themselves into a unique position in our world-view. On the one hand, as we become smokers, our sense of security is boosted by our acceptance into a self-congratulatory social group. At the same time our need to strike out on our own is also appeased as we fly in the face of health-advice and rebel against the wishes of our doctors, teachers and parents. We each become a 'unique' sheep among the flock.

Unfortunately the joke is on us, since we are subscribing to an illusion which when exposed reveals our cool insiders' club to be a misguided cul-de-sac of collective self-delusion.

The world-view of smoking and nicotine is probably the greatest and most difficult aspect of the overall situation to overcome. Most of us who smoke believe that we are at least getting something out of it, and when asked, we will tell other people who have not yet smoked, that they can expect to experience these benefits. Take note that the tobacco or e-cigarette industries never actually promotes any of these theoretical benefits, not wishing to place themselves in a

63

compromised legal position by infringing trade description laws. Luckily for these industries, there is no need to promote illusory benefits, since the smoking population does that for them, from within the prison of their own illusory reality.

Psychologically, most of us are already addicted before we have even inhaled our first cigarette or vape, simply by virtue of the fact that we want to do it. The psychological side is so powerful that it is possible to build up enough preconceived relief from smoking simply through what you are told by the smoking population and the media, that we really can experience psychological relief right from the first cigarette, as I did myself. That is to say the relief feels real, emotionally speaking, but it is not as a direct physical result of the tobacco, but of the fulfilled craving of the ego. Even worse, passive inhaling of tobacco smoke on a regular basis over even a short period of time is sufficient to activate the physical dependency gradually without even having to smoke, so that 'getting into it' can be made much easier.

Take a person, however, who has lived all their life in isolation and has never experienced the concept of smoking, and get them to inhale a cigarette, and I guarantee you their response will be entirely negative. If you simply ask them "Would you like another one?" I can promise you that their answer will be 'No'

So, relative to the illusory world of the smoker, smoking of course does make you a 'cooler' person, but on the greater scheme of things, it really just makes a victim of you. A smoker is a person who is the victim of a fantastic confidence trick on a global scale, and lacks any actual understanding of their real situation, deserving compassion and assistance to emerge from the grip of their own cruelly hijacked ego.

The triggers that lead to our consumption of nicotine are to a great extent a product of social considerations although obviously they vary according to the individual.

Because the addiction is tied in with our basic state of being, the triggers tend to become associated both with situations which we enjoy, because we feel a need to enhance them, and situations which upset us, because we feel that we need some help. What we are told to expect by other smokers has some considerable influence, as do images of smoking in film and television. We are told that it is nice to smoke a cigarette after meals; so when we arrive at the end of a meal, we automatically desire a cigarette. Since the addiction has been triggered and fulfilled, the cigarette that is smoked after the meal is obviously pleasant, and we are nearer to a state of normality, so we feel more at ease. Relative to the world of the addict, we have become a more complete person as a result of the cigarette, and as such we are obviously better equipped to enjoy the post-eating sensation.

We are therefore naturally inclined to do the

same thing every mealtime and to tell others how nice it is too, thus further reinforcing the collective view on post-dinner cigarettes. And so the machine rolls on.

You do not enjoy a situation more because of smoking, rather you need to smoke to be able to enjoy the situation normally. Constant smoking has made you less able to enjoy anything!

Smoking becomes like a 'sacred' ritual, a central focus of your life. This is not surprising since once you are addicted to it, you are dependent on it to feel 'alive'. It can easily come to feel sacred, because your life is sacred.

In all honesty, nicotine will rise to pretty much any occasion you might care to associate it with. Anything, which you choose to associate with nicotine, will become an aspect of your experience of the consumption of nicotine. It is like a chameleon, which adopts the shape of things that it is actually depriving you of. It attaches itself to your life, masquerading as an aid to the processes of living which it is actually making harder.

Because we feel that tobacco, or e-cigarettes, are helping us, we consume them to deal with situations in which our ability to cope feels diminished. Since smoking the cigarette results in our addiction being satisfied, we wind up feeling more capable of dealing with the situation. We move closer to a state of normality.

Since we have fulfilled our addiction in response to the demands of a situation, we associate the cigarette with it. We endow the cigarette or vape with the ability to help us deal with the situation.

Nicotine is not helping us to deal with any situation. It is the nicotine that has actually made us feel that we need help in the first place. We tend to feel that when we stop smoking, a hole will be left in our life, but there was never a hole in the first place. Nicotine gradually created its own hole, which, in its absence, will simply be filled by life.

Prolonged smoking has made us less able to cope with life in general. It not only steals from us the ability to operate efficiently, but it even falsely takes the credit for helping us to operate more efficiently!

The important thing to realise, of course, is that when you look to nicotine to enhance a situation that you are enjoying, or to help you in a situation that you are not enjoying, you would be either enjoying the former situation more or needing less help in the latter if you were not generally way below your peak as a result of the nicotine in the first place!

So, let's look at our FOR/AGAINST list again.

AGAINST:

A significant chance of dying from it.

Costs lots of money.

Prevents you from experiencing what it feels like to be a normal healthy person.

Doesn't actually do anything anyway; apart from make you feel worse than you are supposed to.

FOR:

. . .

Well, as we can see, there are actually no reasons to smoke, so we are effectively saying:
"I take a chance of dying, spend loads of money and miss out on knowing the benefits of simply being what I am, so that I can feel a bit worse than I'm supposed to all of the time."

12

SMOKING AT TIMES OF CRISIS

"I understand all this stuff. I stopped smoking for two years completely, and yes, I did feel like I'd never smoke again and I did feel much better, so I do understand the point you're making. In the end it was just when things got really tough – a close relative had died and my partner had left me and I just thought 'To hell with it, I'm going to smoke a cigarette', and I did. I bought a pack of 20 and I've been smoking ever since. So yes, I understand how much better you feel, and how free you feel, but I simply choose to smoke because I enjoy it and it helps when things get really tough."

The sad fact is that this person has effectively never stopped smoking. Not in the sense of having been rid of the hold that smoking has over them. They stopped, they felt better, but in the end, they started again because they had never really moved beyond the 'smoker's mindset'. This person believes that they enjoy smoking. They have not seen the bigger picture. Deeply rooted in their psyche is the incorrect but ingrained notion that smoking is some kind of 'forbidden fruit'. It is seen as something really bad for you, yes, but ultimately something which can really help you out in times of crisis. The whole of the time that this person stopped smoking, they completely failed to understand the basic fact: smoking has zero benefit and some considerable non-benefit.

The trouble is that as smokers, in the grip of our addicted egos, we believe that we have a reasonable understanding of smoking. This is ridiculous and utterly incorrect.

Nan-in, a Japanese master during the Meiji era (1868–1912), received a university professor who came to inquire about Zen.

Nan-in served tea. He poured his visitor's cup full, and then kept on pouring. The professor watched the overflow until he no longer could restrain himself. "It is overfull. No more will go in!"

"Like this cup," Nan-in said, "you are full of your own opinions and speculations. How can I show you Zen unless you first empty your cup?"

13

STOPPING SMOKING VS. TRANSCENDING THE ADDICTION

If you stop smoking but maintain the illusion that smoking was something from which you derived some kind of benefit, then you have effectively never stopped smoking, and starting again will be as natural as if you had never stopped. Additionally, because you never overcome the illusion that smoking is helping you, you will never experience the true peace of mind that comes from totally transcending the addiction. When you stop you will obviously experience the resultant improvement in physical health from not smoking, but failing to resolve the psychological aspect leaves you still bound by the chains of addiction. The idea that because you stopped smoking once for some time, you understand nicotine addiction, is the voice of the addiction, not of a rational unhindered intelligence.

The fact is that when you really understand smoking, then stopping is simply not the same as when you don't fully understand. Usually we decide, "I am now going to try and stop smoking". On an immediate level, simply making the decision causes so much stress at the fear of the empty world without cigarettes, that the urge to smoke is instantly triggered. Even thinking about trying to stop smoking makes you smoke more!

So, let us imagine that you have finally managed to arrive at a point where you are thinking, "Right, this is it – I am giving up now – I am not smoking any more". Onwards you stride into life, fine for a while until some habitual trigger occurs, such as a moment of crisis. You register the stress, and your subconscious reaction as usual inclines you towards ingesting some nicotine to combat the stress. This triggers your physical addiction, so that you also start to feel awkward, yearning for the physical sensation of a dose of nicotine. However, you can't have one, because you are giving up! A time of stress, but you can't ease it by smoking because you are trying to stop smoking! Naturally you rapidly become more stressed. Immediately your subconscious registers the new stress and sends out more signals that you want nicotine, but you can't have any because you are still trying to give up, so you become more stressed, and so on! Sound familiar? Take another look at fig.3, which illustrates this situation. This is what happens when someone tries to give up by willpower alone, without total understanding. I'm not saying that the person in this situation cannot manage to stop smoking. Of course, many people do manage to muster great personal strength and stop this way. There is a world of difference, though, between stopping smoking or vaping, and transcending nicotine addiction. People who stop this way do often go for long periods of time without smoking.

Many of them forget almost entirely about smoking, but instinctively they still recall the basic smoking 'hit' as something, which, despite all its negative sides, gave them some positive assistance in their life. It is impossible to understand how it feels to be a non-smoker in this way. It does not matter how long you stop for, if you never really understand the nature of the thing you are leaving behind, you will never truly leave it behind. It is a tragic fate to end up this way.

It is as though someone has, for instance, left behind an old friend that they miss. They get used to the new world without the friend - there are many new friends and life has become more positive. In the back of their mind, however, there is a twinge of regret for that lost friend. They move on through life, never realising that the friend is actually there all the time, they have simply made a change in their appearance.

Such is the case with nicotine in that if you miss it then you are missing being in need of something, whereas you are actually in possession of the thing you are missing, in greater quantity and by a more natural route. You not only still possess the thing you are missing, but now have it constantly rather than in measured bursts. Your own wholeness is the commodity that nicotine gives the illusion it is providing you with, whilst making you 'un-whole' through its usage. Only lack of actual understanding prevents you from experiencing this fully.

To feel sentimental about the loss of smoking from your life is to dwell upon a time when you were less than you should be, rather than looking to a future at your full capacity.

14

THE CYNIC WITHIN

When someone who smokes claims to understand or not have a problem with smoking, think of them like this:

Imagine a person standing stationary with a huge rock plummeting directly towards them from a great height. You are shouting at the person "Look out! Move; you are going to be crushed by that falling rock!" The person is smiling at you and nodding their head, replying, "Yes, it's all right, I know", but they remain standing in the same position. The person believes that they have understood you, but obviously they have not, because if they really understood you then they would move out of the way of the rock.

"Well maybe they just want to be squashed by the rock."

If this response occurred to you, then stop and think for a second. As you read this book, observe your conscious reactions to the points raised. The little voice, which often interjects a cynical response in your mind, is the voice of the addiction. It is a part of you, but it is also something independent of you, in that you at your full potential, unbound from nicotine addiction, are a far less cynical being. The addict within is someone whose world is built on false foundations.

Bang ! Bang!

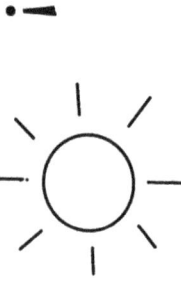

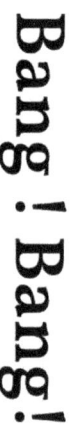

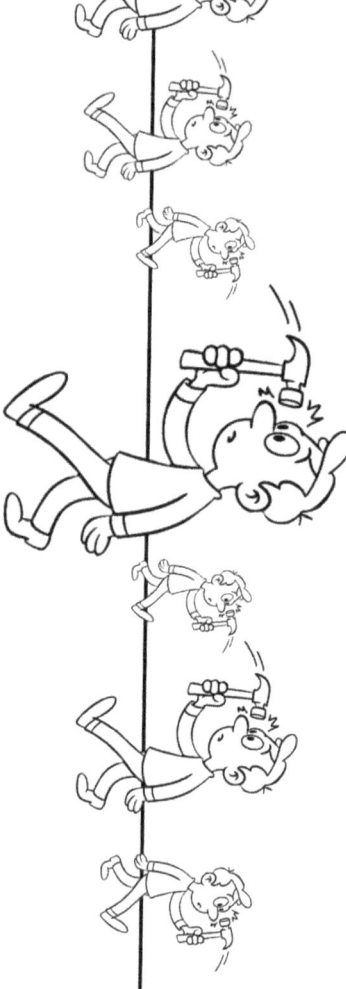

"I'm only doing it because it's my birthday!"

The person created by the union of human and nicotine is a soul in bondage, held in a cage of contradiction.

We all have a natural instinct for self-preservation. We have an inclination towards creating improvement in our situation at any given time. We like to have nice things happen to us as often as possible. The pursuit of satisfaction is an essential aspect of our conscious being.

When we become smokers, then, we become a being at odds with ourselves. It is as though we are walking around hitting ourselves in the face with a hammer, and convincing ourselves we are enjoying it. We are performing a totally meaningless activity because we are misinformed about the real nature of what we are doing. The kind of negative, irrational thinking which gives rise to the above response, or tries to excuse smoking as a product of some kind of in-built self-destructive streak, is thinking born of banging one's head against a brick wall.

Yes, obviously some people do seek self-destruction, but someone who lacks the commitment and inspiration to come up with a more effective or creative form of self-destruction than smoking is hard to take seriously.

Unless someone is genuinely suicidal, the excuse that smoking is born out of a desire for self-harm holds no credence. This idea is a construct of the addicted mind to support its condition. It is not a normal state of mind, needing to constantly justify a considerable level of completely pointless self-injury. To accommodate such irrational behaviour, we will construct almost any excuse. When we are the victims of an addiction, we are essentially a being at odds with ourselves. We are split between the addicted lower self and the unattached truthful higher self. We are divided, and this is something we find hard to accept, which is why we construct reasons such as self-destructiveness to appease our sense of integrity. We do not like to think of ourselves as being split, so we would even rather believe that we are simply self-destructive, because at least endowing ourselves with this negative trait leaves us with a whole personality in terms of our self-image, albeit a somewhat negative one. "I am damaging myself regularly by smoking but that's ok because I am self-destructive." sits far easier with our sense of integrity than "I am damaging myself regularly by smoking and I am an intelligent person who is concerned with my own well-being." The former can be perceived as some kind of coherent argument, the nature of the individual excusing the self-harm; the latter, however, which is also the actual state of most of us as smokers, is essentially nonsensical, and is the simple truth upon which the addicted eye is so reluctant to focus.

You must decide who you really are. Are you really someone who seeks self-destruction? The fact is that if you were a sincerely self-destructive person, then you certainly wouldn't be reading a book designed to help you give up smoking. The very nature of 'wanting' usually implies a sense of desire for something that will make a person feel better than they do at the moment. It inherently suggests a desire for improvement. The nature of 'self-destruction' is to do harm to oneself, i.e. to make one's situation worse than it already is. Therefore to say that you 'want' to smoke because you have a 'self-destructive streak' is something of a contradiction in terms. Foggy meaninglessness is what we find at the heart of nicotine addiction. It is a false world, a house of cards, a world of people who walk around all day banging hammers against their faces. When we try to stop smoking by 'cutting down', or when we stop sentimentally, missing the tobacco as we would a dear friend, then effectively we are saying "Well, I used to hit myself in the face with a hammer up to 40 times a day, but now I only do it once or twice, (or) now I only hit myself on my birthday or at Christmas!" **Nicotine addiction means living in a nonsensical world. An alternate dimension built on false foundations.**

We have discussed how a person can stop smoking cigarettes but remain a nicotine addict, because they have not fully understood the nature of smoking. It is also important to realise that if a person has understood fully, then provided they physically stop smoking, the psychological aspect of the addiction cannot continue to manifest itself.

Sometimes someone may come to realise the truth about smoking, but not immediately 'feel' it. They can see that smoking does not actually do what they thought it did, and that with this knowledge, smoking should become meaningless to them, but they may still feel an irrational desire for tobacco, and therefore be unsure as to whether they can stop smoking. It is possible to recognise that the simple facts about smoking suggest that it should be easy to stop, and yet feel that despite these facts, stopping still seems difficult.

Imagine a person you are aware of but have had little interaction with. You have been told that they have some negative personality traits, but you have not experienced them for yourself. From this position, you can only theorise about them. You can label them as having negative traits, but without direct experience, you cannot really be aware of their personality. You do know that this person theoretically possesses these traits, but without direct experience you do not naturally take account of them in your daily life.

If you spend time with them, however, and gain for yourself experience of their negative side, then you actually become aware of the nature of that which you have previously only known from a third party. Similarly, if you can see the truth about nicotine in theory, then provided you remain focused on that truth and do not ingest any more nicotine, then pretty soon you will undoubtedly come to 'feel' the truth, and thus to 'be a non-smoker.'

The reason that you do not necessarily feel as it might seem you should, is that you are still under the effects of nicotine and the habits it has ingrained in you. It is still in your system, and because you are in the process of overcoming the addiction, that area of yourself feels threatened. The presence of nicotine in your bloodstream has a negative effect upon the functioning of your brain, in exactly the same way that water in petrol would obviously have a negative effect on the functioning of an engine. It helps to reinforce the illusions that enable you to smoke. Because it is destructive to your entire system, your thought processes themselves are not functioning at full capacity. Your physical pangs and basic instinct to smoke are like a fog over your mind. Because you are starting to see the truth, your addicted system reacts with shock to the new realisation and can make it difficult to focus on what is really important. You can see, if you calm your mind, step back and take a really clear look at the situation.

This is a classic illustration of the difference between the 'higher and lower self', in terms of consciousness. The philosophical concept of the 'higher self' refers to the more insightful aspect of ourselves which seems to suggest a more positive and beneficial course of action at any given time. The 'lower self' is that which inclines us towards behaviour that is unconstructive and is mostly driven by the ego in its quest for sense gratification.

A scholar of eastern wisdom might equate the lower self with the mind and the higher self with the soul. One might simply view the higher self as the area of your consciousness that tends to suggest a more intuitive inclination. I'm sure we have all been in situations when we did something we regretted. Probably there was a moment of choice, and we chose the path that made things worse than they were. More often than not in these situations, one can look back and think "I knew I shouldn't do that!" The 'I' that knew we shouldn't do it is the higher self, the aspect of you that always really knows best.

'You', the 'higher' self, can see the simple truth that there is obviously no reason to carry on smoking, and of course many reasons why you shouldn't carry on! The 'lower' self is the part of you that stoically refuses to look on the bright side in spite of the facts; or even in fact paints what is in reality the bright side, as the dark side.

"Oh no. It seems as though I'll just have to stop smoking then, since it doesn't actually do anything anyway. I suppose I'll just feel loads better all the time. I'll not only lose nothing at all, but even finally get the thing I always wanted from smoking, in a permanent way; namely that irresistible sense of being more sorted out, more together and relaxed, which turns out to actually be what it feels like to be a non-smoker. I'm not sure I like the sound of that."

This might seem nonsensical, but I have often seen people say that given that there is obviously no reason to carry on smoking, they are therefore going to stop, and that since they were trying to stop, they have succeeded, but still wear a face of abject gloom. The recovering addict can sometimes seem like a person who has won the jackpot on a quiz show, but is dejectedly unsure whether they might rather keep the loser's consolation prize instead!

Relax! Let yourself off the hook, because that is what you always wanted anyway. Ignore the little voice inside that perpetually says "but..." to every rational argument you throw in front of it.

15

A MATHEMATICAL PERSPECTIVE

This won't mean something to everyone, but for those with mathematical minds, it may be relevant. I want to illustrate the way in which overcoming nicotine addiction is inevitable once you have comprehended a certain amount of real information about it, even if it does not immediately seem so.

When I was in school, I was put into an 'extra maths' class for pupils who were particularly good at mathematics. To be honest, I wasn't really especially good at maths, but I just scraped the right percentage in an exam, so I was enrolled in the class. We studied calculus and co-ordinate geometry. I can't pretend to be an expert in these fields, but something of their basic mechanism has stayed with me, and over the years I have come to see some kind of parallel between co-ordinate geometry and the process by which we transcend nicotine addiction. Co-ordinate geometry is a system of geometry in which points, lines, shapes and surfaces are represented by algebraic expressions. For example, $y=2x+1$ gives a straight line.

Initially, all one possesses are an equation, a series of variables and a blank sheet of paper, or a set of facts, some time to think and one's own consciousness.

Applying each of the variables to the equation, and calculating the results, one arrives at a set of co-ordinates, which enable one to plot a series of points across the paper. Although the course of the points is not initially known, it is predetermined by the specific numeric values of the variables and the results that are therefore unavoidably obtained when they are fed through the equation. Similarly, the facts about nicotine addiction lead unavoidably to the state of consciousness of the non-smoker, since they completely invalidate the entire smoking concept.

As the course of the graph is initially invisible, so the results of understanding nicotine addiction are not initially apparent. The facts may seem to be pointing in a direction, but at the same time, one may still feel tempted to smoke, or one may make a few calculations and plot a few points, but not yet see the full image on the paper. The full image will ultimately come into view, however, irrespective of personal speculation upon its outcome, provided one keeps making the calculations. Similarly, the truth, with all the implications that its full realization entails, will certainly dawn once one is in possession of the facts, provided one keeps thinking about them. Thinking about nicotine addiction is as inevitable as the processes of the addiction itself. It doesn't actually matter how much the addiction kicks and screams within you, your own natural reasoning process, given the full facts of the situation, will inevitably dismantle the smoking myth irretrievably at some point along the course of the graph of your life. It is a mathematical certainty:

1+1=2
truth + understanding = conclusion

16

A Visualisation

Imagine a person who is unaffected by illusions.

This person has a completely clear grasp of everything they encounter.

This person is unaffected by the illusions which surround smoking.

Imagine that this person comes upon smoking in complete awareness of the facts. They know that smoking is something that will have no beneficial effect on them whatsoever. They also know that if they decide to use tobacco or e-cigarettes anyway, it will in addition to not providing them with any benefits, have numerous negative effects.

Imagine how this person will feel about smoking as a whole.

They will view it with no interest whatsoever. If it interests them in any way, it will be simply that they are fascinated by how anyone could possibly do anything so pointless.

There is obviously no way that this person would smoke.

Imagine that you are this person. Imagine how it would feel to fully understand that smoking quite simply does not do anything. Imagine how it would feel to understand exactly how the illusion that smoking feels good comes about. Imagine how easy it would be not to smoke if you were this person. The point is that if you can imagine how it would feel to be this person, you are this person.

If you can see this, if you have the capacity to imagine yourself in a state of complete understanding of nicotine addiction, then obviously some portion of yourself does genuinely understand. You can make the choice to focus on that area of yourself rather than one which would have you blindly injuring yourself for completely illusory reasons.

17

THE MOST ADDICTIVE SUBSTANCE

Imagine I offer you a pill. It is the most addictive substance known to humankind. All it will actually do to you is to make you feel worse than you would usually do. But, after a period of taking these pills, they will start to create the illusion that they are actually making you feel better, because you will need them to feel anywhere near normal. Then, once you are addicted, you will never feel normal again while the addiction lasts, and you will become less and less healthy, and even stand an increasing chance of dying through their use.

Would you like one?

Could I possibly persuade you to take one?

No, of course I could not. It is extremely unlikely that I could persuade you to take one of those pills, or that you could persuade anyone else to. Try it. Try making the same offer to anyone. Try to persuade them. I don't think you could do it. No one in their right mind would think about taking one of these pills. Not only that, but saying 'No' to one would be a really easy thing to do. Going on the description above, it is hard to see any reason why anyone would think about taking one of these pills.

The pills are exactly the same as cigarettes.

So how, then, could you possibly ever smoke again?

"But...."

But nothing. And more importantly – why say "But," at all? Why would you? Think about it. Why would you possibly spend any time whatsoever trying to think of a reason why you might take one of these pills?

Having discovered that your tea has been spat in, and that you have perfectly good tea, why would you try to find any reason why you would still drink the tea with someone else's spit in it?

If you discover that you have been doing something, which turns out to be disadvantageous to you, you obviously stop doing it.

"But it's just not as simple as that!"

Why isn't it as simple as that?

If you discovered that you had been accidentally taking these pills for a while, thinking that they did something else, what would you do?

You would immediately stop taking them.

It is very straightforward. The pill is a very easy thing to understand. All they do is to make you feel worse than you should. After a while, you will develop a dependency on them so that you will need them to feel anywhere near normal. Without correct information, this situation could be misinterpreted as the pills actually making you feel good, but this is obviously not the case. While you are taking them, you will run the risk of dying through their use, and to add insult to injury, they will even cost you money! They are an entirely unappealing prospect. You really couldn't possibly consider taking them under any circumstances.

Really think about this clearly and carefully. Don't let your mind scan over this. Think about the pill that I am describing. Think carefully about every detail of what it does. Really perceive it as a product, with all the properties that I have outlined. Really try to imagine any reason why you might want to start taking them. There is simply no way you could or would do it.

Do you understand what the pill I am describing does?

It's pretty straightforward. Not too much to understand. It is an entirely negative thing. There is absolutely no reason to take them.

You know that if I presented you with one of these pills right now, you would not have any interest in taking it.

The only difference between the pill and the cigarette is the way that they look. The pill is the cigarette, so given that you understand the pill, you are obviously not going to smoke any more cigarettes!

Are you sure that you will never smoke any more cigarettes?

If you are not sure, why not?

What is there to be unsure about?

If you can see that the pill is obviously something you would not entertain taking, then how could you ever consider smoking again?

If you feel that you could consider smoking again, then step outside yourself and take a look at the contradiction that is happening here. You can see that the pill is something you would not touch and yet perhaps you are not sure that you will never smoke again, but they are fundamentally the same thing!

Which you are you?

Why would you want to carry on doing something when the driving force behind you doing it is a desire for something that will be fulfilled by not doing it?! Why would you want to do something, which is entirely bad for you?

"Look, I know it's bad for me, but I still enjoy doing it."

Yes, relative to each cigarette you smoke, you do enjoy it, but what is the nature of the enjoyment? As we have discussed, the thing that you enjoy is the sensation of being 'more sorted out' that you experience when you smoke. But what is that experience? It is your climb back to the state that you would occupy all the time if you were a non-smoker! The reason that the cigarettes or vapes make you feel good is that the nicotine you are ingesting as a result of smoking has enslaved your system. You need the nicotine to feel normal. Therefore when you smoke, you are fulfilling a need that your system has developed. When you smoke, you feed the thing upon which your whole sense of well-being depends. You satisfy the addiction, and so your state of being moves back towards its normal level, i.e. better than you did before smoking the cigarette.

The point is that if the cigarette makes you feel good, then that is not the effect of tobacco or nicotine. It is the effect of climbing back towards your optimum capacity. The way that you felt before you smoked the cigarette was not normality. If you smoke, then the way you feel as you move through an average day is worse than the way a typical non-smoker feels. When you are a smoker, you spend the whole of your time with your nervous system saturated with a highly toxic carcinogenic poison. You cannot possibly imagine that you ever feel anywhere near normal under these circumstances.

Remember, if you stopped smoking before, but later started again, do not assume that you understand how a non-smoker feels. The feeling of being a non-smoker is a product of more than simply being someone who does not physically smoke. I use the term 'non-smoker' to mean someone who not only does not smoke, but also knows that they will never smoke.

There really are so many potential differences in perception of something depending on how we regard it. To say that someone 'knows that they will never smoke' can mean very different things.

You might see this person as someone very strong who has resolved never to smoke again. They have absolutely decided that is the end of it. They will never smoke again. They may be tempted, or maybe they only catch a breath of tobacco smoke occasionally and think a little wistfully of their smoking days, but they are strong and determined.

They will never smoke again. This person still has quite a bit to occupy themselves with, though. True, they will never smoke again, so in one sense they have succeeded. If they have had to act determinedly to achieve this goal, though, then they are still fighting themselves.

If you have to leave smoking behind with any sense of loss, then you are not leaving it behind at all. If you are going to miss smoking then you might as well smoke, for all the psychological good stopping is going to do you. If you have any feeling of loss, then you have not understood. To feel a valid sense of loss, one must lose something. The reality of stopping smoking is that you lose nothing.

The one element of smoking which you hold dear, the rush of completeness that you get from the best cigarette of the day, is actually what it feels like to be a non-smoker. There is no loss.

Imagine then the person who 'knows that they will never smoke' again, but knows it in the same way that they know they will never deliberately walk into walls. It is not difficult for that person to deal with the knowledge that they will never walk into a wall.

Not smoking once you have understood the nature of smoking will not be a matter of stress to you. How could it?

Look at figs 2,3 and 4 again (pages 47,48 and 49). The situation is really very clear. In fig.3, you can see how stress snowballs when we try to stop by willpower alone. In fig.4, we can see how understanding of the situation diffuses the stress. As we have discussed, the stress from stopping smoking is mostly caused by misinformation about smoking itself. Stopping smoking is purely a matter of being aware of the facts.

If you are genuinely aware of the facts then you are a non-smoker.

"What at this moment is lacking?"

Master Rinzai

18

AMENDING YOUR BEHAVIOUR

Imagine person A who lives in the country. Person A goes to visit person B. Person B tells person A "Look at this excellent plant. If you eat it, it will improve your health," Person A starts eating the plant on a daily basis. After a while, person A starts experiencing stomach pains. They go to a doctor, who asks about their diet. When the plant is mentioned, the doctor exclaims, "Oh no, you don't eat that do you? That plant is actually really bad for you. People used to think that it was good for you, but research has shown it is a really bad plant to eat. That is what is causing your pains."

Person A stops eating the plant.

Person A feels better.

Person A does not 'forget' or 'slip up' and start eating the plant again. They know that it is bad for them.

Person A was under an illusion about something, but in the light of new information, they are now proceeding comfortably, free of their illusion, and consequently feeling much better. True, they had probably got into the habit of eating the plant every day, and they will probably see the plant growing around the area, or meet other less well-informed people who eat it, but now that they actually know the real situation, it will not be difficult to live without it.

You thought that smoking did something. It doesn't. It does something else. You had information that was not correct. Now you have information that is correct.

In the light of new information about something, we amend our thinking and behaviour to accommodate the new information.

Obviously, you don't smoke then.

Luckily for you, not only do you simply stop doing something negative, but all the things you thought you would lose by stopping are actually things you will finally attain by stopping.

They are simply feelings of greater togetherness, which are the permanent state of the non-smoker.

So you see there really is no 'giving up smoking'. There is simply clear understanding.

For example, I once saw a small child trying to eat rabbit droppings. The child did not understand. At this point, the child was someone who voluntarily ate shit. At some point, the child's parent succeeded in making the child aware of the nature of rabbit shit. From that moment on, the child was no longer someone who ate shit. They had simply come to understand a mistake that they had been making, and consequently amended their behaviour accordingly. It is unlikely that the child ever ate shit again.

You are a person who has become addicted to

a drug. You are aware that the drug is damaging to your health, but you choose to use it anyway, because of the sensation you get from it. It calms you down, helps you to relax, makes you feel more 'together' etc. You enjoy the effects of the drug, and they seem to outweigh the adverse health considerations.

You have made a mistake. It is not your fault. It was an easy mistake to make. There was little or no real information made available to you. You were given the impression that you were aware of all the facts. You were told that smoking was bad for you, but you were also given the impression that you would experience some positive effects as well. You were made to feel as though you were making a balanced decision to take the risk to your health in favour of the benefits that smoking affords you. Every other smoker you spoke to would tell you of the advantages of smoking – how nice it is to have that little relaxing prop. Once you had 'got into' smoking, it did seem to start to fulfil its promise. Little by little, you came to experience more pleasant effects from its consumption.

Tobacco and nicotine do not do what you thought they did. The positive sensation ('the rush') that you experience from smoking is actually how you are supposed to feel all of the time. Imagine that best cigarette of the day. Imagine that first inhale. Imagine how good you feel at the peak of that – the smoke held in your lungs for a moment, as your state of being resolves itself, a sense of calm and satisfaction settling over you. Realise and acknowledge how good that feels. That feeling is how I feel all the time, me and all the other non-smokers. Honest! I used to smoke for years. I have no reason to lie to you. It really is this simple. Your system has become dependent on nicotine. You need it to feel normal.

The amazing feeling, that you get from a 'nicotine hit' is not caused by the nicotine. It is the sensation of your nicotine-dependent system receiving a 'fix' – a dose of nicotine to fulfil the need created by your addiction. It is the sensation of your system moving towards a state of normality. It only feels amazing because real life feels amazing. To be human and healthy feels amazing. The peak of the 'nicotine rush' is the world of the non-smoker. When you smoke you receive it only in occasional measured bursts. When you are a non-smoker, you receive it constantly. It is the same thing.

19

INTO THE LIGHT

A smoker is like a person who sits in a room in darkness. Every time they smoke a cigarette, the curtains open and they are able to look out at a beautiful sunny field outside, with people playing and sunbathing happily. Then the curtains close

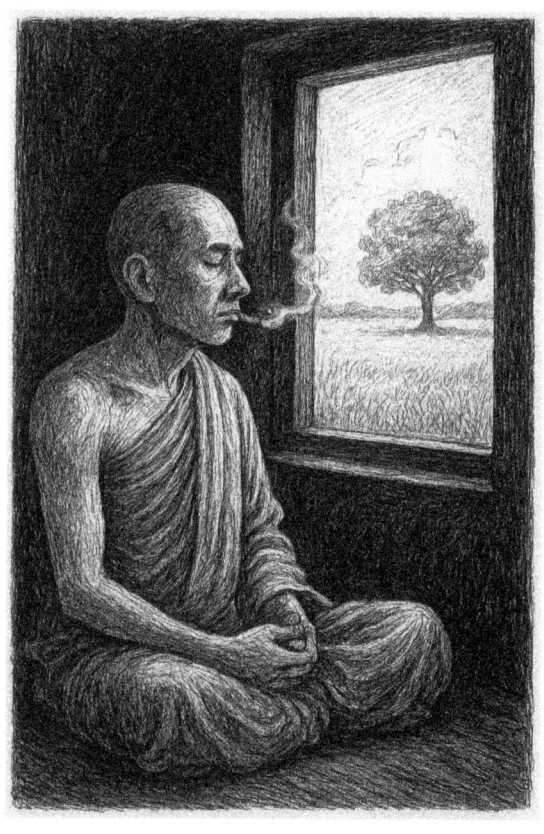

again and the room is plunged back into darkness until the next cigarette. The smoker is quite happy with this situation, accepting it as normal and even remarking enthusiastically on the nice view they get to look at whenever the curtains open. What they fail to realise, however, is that if they simply stop smoking altogether, pretty soon the room itself will disappear, leaving them sitting outside in the field with everyone else.

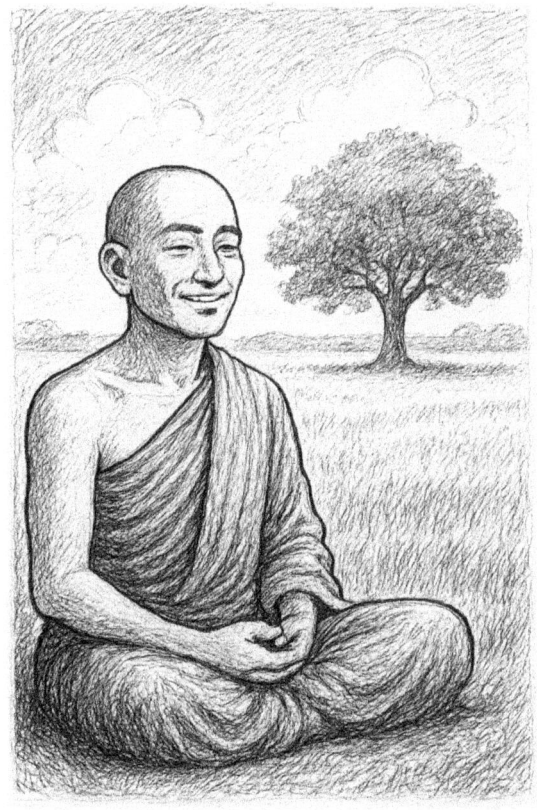

Tobacco becomes like a candle at which you are staring. As you stare at the flame for longer and longer, it appears that you are gradually heading into darkness, and that the candle flame stands as your light in that darkness. However, you are not really heading into darkness, it only seems that way because you have been staring at the flame for so long that your surroundings have come to seem dark by comparison. If you blow out the candle, however, you will discover that you are surrounded by light.

When you smoke, it feels as though you feel normal most of the time, and when you smoke a cigarette, it makes you feel a little better. This is an illusion. Yes, when you smoke a cigarette, you do feel better, but only because the nicotine that has been eating into your nervous system has made you feel much worse than you are supposed to in the first place. Nicotine gives the impression that it is pulling you up, but conversely nicotine is actually the thing that has dragged you down to the depths. And in that simple truth lies the core dynamic of addiction.

You are addicted to it, so that if you don't have it, you will feel bad, and when you get it you will be fulfilled, and so feel nearer to how you would be if you didn't smoke at all.

If you stop smoking, all that will happen is that you will recover. If you have tried to stop before, but it has been too difficult, do not be disheartened. It will be different this time. If you understand, then stopping is easy. You just have to think very clearly and understand. If you are genuinely aware of the facts then you cannot smoke.

Of course, when I say that you 'cannot' carry on smoking, I do not mean to sound as though I am forbidding you to do something. Of course you can carry on smoking if you want to, but let's be honest - why would anyone want to spend time doing something which is entirely negative? If there were some reason, then I would understand.

"I enjoy it. That's reason enough."
The thing that you are enjoying is the sensation of being a non-smoker! The feeling that you enjoy so much is the nearest that you can come, as a smoker, to feeling normal, and it still falls short of how normality actually feels. The fact that you enjoy it is exactly the reason why you should stop doing it.

If you derive any pleasure from smoking, then the amount of pleasure is the measure of how far from normal you are feeling the rest of the time!

If you take any pleasure in smoking then ask yourself this question:

Would it not be much nicer to feel this sort of pleasure more strongly and all of the time rather than simply when I smoke a cigarette?
The fact that you want to carry on smoking in order to feel the pleasurable effect that you

get from it is perfectly natural. You are bound to desire this feeling because it is as natural to you as breathing. The effect you are feeling is what you are naturally supposed to feel like all of the time. It is not supposed to be a feeling that you get from cigarettes or vapes. The only reason that cigarettes and vapes appear to make you feel like this is that you are dependent on them to help you to feel normal, so when you smoke one, because you basically feel way below normal, they appear to make you feel better.

The dose of nicotine fulfils the desire created by your system's dependency. Your addiction is fuelled. You move back towards normality. Normality is a naturally pleasant state, therefore you feel better than you did before smoking the cigarette.

The point is that the enjoyment is entirely illusory, since the less enjoyable state from which you came is one that has been created by the use of nicotine in the first place. The net effect of nicotine is that it causes more damage than a 'nicotine fix' appears to repair.

What nicotine takes from you is the feeling of being alive. Because the drug is very slowly killing you, the feeling you get from a nicotine fix is totally fundamental. It is an all-encompassing sense of well-being - the feeling of being alive. Smoking cigarettes and inhaling vapes make you feel more alive, because that is exactly what they are stealing from you. It is like a cruel taunt: a carrot on a stick. When you smoke, the momentary rush of well-being you experience is a bitter irony. We cling to that prop with all our might, never realising that the thing to which we cling is in actuality what we would receive in abundance if we would only let go!

20

Acknowledge the Dark Side!

To truly transcend nicotine addiction, you must identify the personality of the addiction, which resides within you. The addiction is a selfish, cunning entity, which since you live with it for so long, you come to accommodate as part of yourself. It will go to any lengths to justify and maintain its existence. It manipulates you through your ego. You come to mistake its shortcomings for your own.

Obviously it is a part of you, but the addiction takes the form of a kind of "sub-personality" within you, accentuating your lesser personality traits. It is the voice that stoically pipes up "But..." long past the point where all arguments have been won. The nicotine addiction itself is the entity that would have you happily drinking tea with someone else's saliva in it for the rest of your days and laughs behind your back while you are doing it.

If you find this hard to accept, consider this: when one member of a group of smokers decides that they want to give up, more often than not, the other smokers will persistently offer cigarettes to the individual who is trying to give up. As the person attempting to stop smoking, you will probably be subjected to a fairly constant barrage of "go on, have one - you know you want to!" and other such taunts, especially in group situations. What does this say about the other people in the group - the ones who still smoke? If your friend, someone you love, is trying to free themselves from something that is hurting them, why on earth would you possibly try in any way to persuade them to carry on doing the thing they are trying to escape from?!

Think about it — it is really sinister. I remember doing it myself. I am not proud of it now, but at the same time I forgive myself, because I was not in control of my actions. If you can find it in yourself to try to hinder someone you love from helping themselves, then take a very good look at yourself. Are you really like this? Are you honestly the kind of person who would wish harm upon a loved one? Don't be tempted to dismiss this as a matter of little consequence. Let's be honest about this — thousands of people die every day from smoking related illness.

Obviously, smokers do this because as addicts, we cannot stand to see someone conquer the thing that defeats us. When a member of a group of smokers stops smoking, the addict within each other member of the group begins to panic and a selfish personality rears its head.

This is not the real you. Your higher self is not a selfish person. The part of you that would have your loved ones harm themselves, for the sake of your own bruised ego is not a part of yourself that you can call a friend. This is the personality of the addiction, fuelled by the nicotine in your bloodstream, and if it can make you behave in this way, then what does that say about nicotine?

It is easy to laugh off the above example with the same light heartedness with which we screen ourselves from embracing the real nature of the smoking menace. But have no doubt, no matter how insignificant tobacco and/or nicotine may seem in the average day of a smoker, the fact remains that smoking is one of the biggest causes of death to the human species. It is also one of the biggest industries on earth. Nicotine is not your friend. Your body is your friend – do it a favour.

So how do you feel then?

Are you ready to try to give up smoking/vaping?

This is of course a meaningless question. It is pointless to think in terms of 'trying to give up' smoking. This implies that you are going to make an effort to surrender something from your life, which was of benefit to you; something positive which will no longer be yours.

Like when people say that they are 'cutting down' on their smoking. Rather than doing something which has a purely negative effect on me twenty times a day, I am going to do it only twice. Rather than hitting myself in the face with a hammer twenty times a day, I am only going to do it once a day at bedtime, or only on a special occasion!

There is no cutting down. There is no deciding that now you are going to try to give up. There is simply an accurate appraisal of the facts of a situation and an appropriate reaction. Rather than thinking in terms of 'giving up smoking', it seems far more appropriate to think in terms of 'dropping' smoking in the same way as one might drop any completely undesirable item such as a burning hot coal. Let it fall away from you without a trace of sentimentality!

Smoking: something that we know to have significant negative effects, but that initially appears to have some beneficial effects. On closer inspection, it reveals itself to be a subtle trick and in fact has only negative effects.

Quite simply then something that we obviously don't do!

Why would we? Why on earth would anyone smoke if they understood it? How could they? It is impossible to comprehend!

"Ah, but that's just me. I'm crazy. I just do these really pointless self-destructive things, even when I know I shouldn't."

The addiction will always have something to say, no matter how completely you have examined the situation. Think about what the little voice inside is actually doing. Imagine a person who for some absurd reason is saying that there is some chance that they will drink tea that has been spat in, because they are crazy and do pointless self-destructive things! This is essentially what the little voice inside that throws up objections, is doing.

You want a cigarette? You want that feeling you get from smoking?

Have it!

But have the real feeling. In other words, give yourself the reality of what it is that you want from smoking - being a non-smoker! Don't deny the desire - understand it. You might say that non-smokers are effectively the only real smokers, in that only the non-smokers actually get what it is that the smokers believe they are getting by smoking. So if you were to define a 'smoker' as 'someone who does something on a regular basis which results in them being calmer, less stressed, more complete, more able to see, hear, taste, smell and feel, then a 'smoker' is someone who does not smoke cigarettes! What is it that they do then, that makes them feel so good?

They live. Pretty simple really, and surprisingly rewarding.

21

BOREDOM

So, have you understood then? I could just keep on and on circling around this. The part of you which keeps on demanding more information is simply the addiction itself, which would always like to make things more complicated than they actually are.

There will never be anything new to say. There will never be any reason to smoke. Once you have seen the truth, there are only reasons to stop. The part of you that keeps saying "but.." is the addiction. You can keep on answering it, but it will never stop asking questions until you decide not to respond to it any more. You can see that there is no reason to carry on smoking. The addiction would have you believe that this is a dismal, upsetting fact, but how could it be?

The reality is that all the things you thought that you were getting from smoking were illusions. It only relieved stress because you were more stressed than you should be as a result of ingesting nicotine. It only tasted good because you needed it to feel normal, so you came to associate the taste with your climb back to normality.

Nicotine is an entirely negative drug. It does nothing for you at all. It makes you feel worse than you are supposed to. It creates the illusion that it is making you feel good because you need it to feel normal.

"Please stop repeating yourself, I know what you are saying and I'm getting really bored of hearing you say it..."

Ok, so you are getting bored of hearing me repeat the basic facts about smoking and nicotine addiction. Presumably that means that you understand them, and that you are finding it boring hearing the same set of phrases repeated needlessly? If that is the case then you are now a newly liberated non-smoker!

Is that true? Are you now taking your first steps into a nicotine-free world?

If so, then congratulations! I know it feels a little strange at first – almost too simple somehow! Be assured, though, that if you really feel that you have got it, then you have. No amount of internal objection can stand in the way once you have made that connection with reality, and it will get easier day by day.

If you are not yet at this point, but were getting bored with my repetitions then think about that response. You are bored with reading the same things repeated over and over. The point is that the things that I am repeating are a set of very simple facts that lead naturally to a simple conclusion. They show in a perfectly straightforward way that there is absolutely no reason to carry on smoking, and that anything you ever wanted from smoking will actually come to you anyway if you stop.

Within the realm of human relationships, one may observe many archetypal patterns that we tend to adopt. One may often look at the relationship dilemmas of one's friends and see reflections of one's own behaviour.

An archetypal relationship situation is that of the lover who is unable to accept the end of a relationship. Kate has left Bill. She finds that the relationship has grown stale. She doesn't really love Bill any more. She wants her independence back.

Bill, on the other hand still loves Kate. Bill thinks that Kate is kidding herself. He thinks that she is deluding herself, and that soon she will realise. Bill keeps trying to make Kate understand. He is getting frustrated with Kate's inability to admit to herself that she really still loves him. It makes him so mad. Why won't she just stop being so stupid and come back to him?!

The truth is, unfortunately for Bill, that Kate simply does not love him anymore. She is never going to come back. She is happy with her new life.

Bill is frustrated with what he perceives as Kate's stubbornness. He makes himself more and more frustrated each time Kate tells him that she is sure that it is really over. In Bill's mind, his frustration is being caused by Kate's refusal to see things his way. As far as he is concerned, Kate is the one who is being frustrating. The reality of the situation is that Bill is frustrating himself by his egocentric refusal to actually look at the real situation and admit that things have changed.

If you are finding my repetitions boring but have not yet grasped the truth of nicotine addiction, then you are Bill, my friend!

The reason that I keep repeating myself is that I know from experience that people do not necessarily immediately understand the real situation, so I circle around it, trying to penetrate the fog of addiction. If you had understood, then what you read would be unlikely to bore you because you would be too busy feeling elated. Either that, or you would have simply stopped reading at the point of understanding, realising that your freedom begins when you decide to really look at yourself, not with the last page of the book. I'm sorry but that is the truth, and only you can choose to see it.

Nicotine addiction is a little like a tangled wood. I can help you through the wood to the gate at the other side, but only you can make the final decision to step through the gate.

One of the best things about this decision, is that to decide to step through conveniently requires you to do absolutely nothing, in much the same way as the person sat in the darkened room gets to sit in the sunny field simply by doing nothing.

Stop punishing yourself!
If you consider the facts, I think you will find that the truth has already made the decision for

you. The only question is how long will you spend arguing with yourself over it. You can deliberate forever, but you are never going to come up with anything new. All you have to do is to rise above the irrational voice within and make a firm decision. Anything that makes you feel as though you should do something totally harmful to yourself for the sake of something that we have established you will never really attain, is not something you should invest any faith in. You are not the addiction. You are a pure being. You can decide. You can exercise your freedom of choice. You can decide that no matter how you may feel emotionally about the issue, the only course of action must be to stop smoking. You can make the absolute decision never to smoke again. You can know that you will never smoke again. You can decide to acknowledge that this is something you know, and in the making of that decision lies your victory.

Once you know that you are taking control, that you are not going to allow any more nicotine into your body, you have won. It does not matter if a part of you still protests – that part will soon fade. It will not be the same as when you have 'tried to stop' before. You did not know the whole situation before. It is the idea that you are leaving something behind that there is some reason to miss, that makes it hard for people to stop smoking.

You know there is nothing to miss. Have faith. Suspend your disbelief. It really is this simple. When you start to heal, you will come to feel strangely similar to how you did right after that best inhale of the day, only constantly rather than just when you smoke a cigarette. I can still remember so vividly the moment it hit me. It was a couple of weeks after I had smoked my last cigarette. I was walking into town from my house. The sun was out and the sky was blue. As I walked I suddenly became aware of a kind of warmth inside me: a glow that seemed to fill me. It was both a physical and an emotional feeling that suffused the whole of my being. I was in an unusually good mood. I seemed to have an extra spring in my step. I was feeling really groovy!

As I registered the feeling, and I latched onto it, affirming that it was real and not only a momentary blip of some kind, it snowballed, and I started laughing with disbelief. I felt as though in some kind of way I had never felt this good. It was as though I had lost some depth of negative feeling from myself: as though my basic capacity to feel bad had been reduced in some way. At the same time, I felt light hearted in a way that I had never known. Except that... it was also familiar - something I had felt before, a long time ago. It was the feeling of being a non-smoker - a combination of physical healing and psychological realisation. Being a clear, normal human being, without the endlessly restless cycle of desire simmering within me. I knew then how it feels to be free. When I physically stopped smoking cigarettes, I had been exhilarated, because I genuinely knew that I would never smoke again. I had still felt weird, though, because the addiction and the nicotine itself were still in my system, so although I knew it was over, it did not fully feel as though it was over. This is what I mean when I say you have to suspend your disbelief. There is a part of you which may have difficulty totally accepting that you are really going to feel any different. You are. How could you not? At a basic level, for the first time in a long time, you are going to stop diluting your bloodstream with a highly toxic chemical! Imagine trying to run a car on petrol mixed with dishwater - it just wouldn't run properly! This is effectively what you have been doing to yourself.

You are actually going to stop. You will no longer contain nicotine, so the physical will no longer support the psychological. Step into the unknown and you will be rewarded for your leap of faith. Focus on the facts rather than the fiction. Keep this book on you for a while to remind you. The more clearly you understand the details of what you have been ensnared by and what you are moving into, the smoother the transition will be.

You can be anything you want if you put your mind to it. For starters why not try simply being yourself. If you smoke cigarettes, or vape, even this fundamental human position is denied to you. Your thoughts are your ongoing discourse with life as it unfolds. Your brain is the organ that processes your thoughts. Your mind is kept alive by the blood, which flows through your body. As a smoker you choose to spend the whole of your time with your bloodstream diluted by a carcinogenic poison. Given this as a basis for your existence, do you seriously think that you can expect to be experiencing anything approaching normality?

It is absolutely crucial for everyone who smokes to fully understand what they are doing. You will know when you really have understood, because you will realise that smoking is over for you. If you still think you might smoke then keep on reading until you understand. Understanding is the key.

If you really understand, then you will not smoke again. Why would anyone, knowing this, choose to smoke?

"Because I'm addicted."

What a 'cop-out' phrase! It is so easy to just write oneself off as an addict – "Oh well I'm addicted, so that's the end of it then. No need to try and figure the whole thing out." What does "addicted" mean? It means that you cannot stop doing something. Why can you not stop smoking? There is no great physical suffering that occurs. The difficulty comes in dealing with the desire. The desire is the product of incorrect information about the nature of smoking. We desire nicotine because to some extent we view it as a positive thing. We have established that the perceived positive aspects of smoking are illusory. Cigarettes and vapes are entirely negative things. There is no reason at all to use them. Any reason that you saw for smoking is false. The things that you thought you were getting were what you will actually get by stopping.

You thought smoking did something. Therefore you smoked.

Oops, made a mistake – it doesn't do what you thought; it does something else, not so good. Therefore you don't smoke.

"When you realise nothing is lacking, the whole world belongs to you."

Lau Tsu

22

BEYOND SMOKING

"Oh no, what a shame! How terrible. What cold empty future awaits me without my nice prop to hold me up? What a terrible thought then, that obviously there is no reason to carry on smoking, and I will just have to heal and recover and come to feel whole and healthy. I will no longer live with the possibility of death from a smoking-related illness, and pay good money to do so. I will miss my lovely secure smoking life."

It is very easy to slip into viewing a nicotine-free future as something negative. If you spend a considerable period of time in a dependency upon something, you naturally come to feel as though the thing upon which you are dependent represents security to you. In reality though, the only security it represents is the security of mental inactivity, since when surrendering to an addiction, one does not really think for oneself. This is the nature of addiction – it makes a horror out of the 'empty' place without the thing to which you are addicted. The reality is always that conversely the state of addiction is the place of horror and the security is something that waits beyond the addiction.

Real security is being at peace with yourself.

Let's take a moment to break addiction as a concept, down into its constituent emotional parts. So firstly, there is a place which is perceived to represent security. A bit like a security blanket. The addicted self assumes this to be the 'known', familiar place – the status quo, where nothing has yet needed to be given up. For the addict, the focus of this (the substance of the security blanket, if you like), is the thing to which the person is attached. This can be nicotine, or alcohol, chocolate, sex, or whatever. So, there is a feeling of security, and there is the perceived source of that feeling.

Next, there is a fear state. Anxiety. Loss. The coldness of the world without the security blanket. The perception is that this is the state that will be the inevitable end result of having to abandon the source of the security state. Without cigarettes or vapes, the world will be cold, uncertain, difficult to manage, etc.

And because of this perception, there is a state of resistance. An instinct to pull back and to not abandon the perceived source of security. A defensiveness that is triggered, when there is any discussion of, or attempt to abandon the perceived source of comfort.

All of these conflicting elements, lead to a stalemate. No motion forwards or backwards is possible. This is pretty much the standard model for all addictions.

And what is causing the problem, the conflict, that keeps people in the addicted condition, is the misassignment of the states of consciousness within the overall scenario, to their perceived sources.

The root of the issue is this pairing of the security state, and the fear state. As long as the person considers the thing to which they are addicted, to be the source of their sense of security, and that therefore having to give it up will inevitably result in the fear state, the longer they will be imprisoned in the stalemate.

If you think about it, 'security', means having your feet on stable ground. Emotionally speaking, you know where you stand. There is food in the cupboard, and the mortgage is paid. Whereas, when one is addicted to something, in reality it is not really what you would call 'secure'; there is a constant swing, between desire for the thing, needing to get hold of the thing, getting hold of the thing, having the thing, feeling briefly fulfilled by the thing, and then not having it again, and cycling back to the desire again. It is actually quite a choppy sea one has to navigate, but nonetheless it is a known quantity, and it has been there for some time, so we label it as security. And we cling to it tightly.

But in actuality, this interpretation of the scenario is incorrect. These misperceptions have been worn-in over a long period of time. So long, that they have come to feel like normality.

If we look at the state beyond the process of giving up the source of the addiction, objectively, all that it actually is, is life without that swing back and forth between desire, fulfilment, loss and desire again. The whole cycle of wanting and needing, and obtaining and wanting again, will not be there. And yet we somehow conclude that this place will be the fear state. Surely that absence of the cycle of desire and fulfilment, sounds like quite a secure place? What is there to fear from not endlessly desiring something that we can never really fulfil? The reason for this misassignment, is that we never really consider actually being free from the addiction in the future, we just focus on the loss of the thing to which we are attached.

So, let's look at that fear state again.

We can't deny that it is a part of the scenario. We feel it. We feel anxiety, as an addict, when we are trying to look at the addiction, but we default to the assumption that it is what awaits us in the future. But yet we are actually experiencing it right now, in the present. The fear state is actually happening, even though we assign it as the future result of having to abandon the security blanket. Even as we look into an empty future without our source of comfort, we are feeling fear, and rather than confront the real nature of that fear, we project it conveniently into the 'unknown' future, where we tell ourselves we won't have to actually deal with it, while we remain wrapped in our blanket. But the fact is that within this flawed evaluation of the situation, we are already in the fear state. And here lies the key to the whole misperception.

The core problem within the status quo of addiction, is the perception that the present moment is secure, and the future beyond the end of addiction is insecure. The reality, is that to be in a constant state of desire that is never really fulfilled, that is doing us no good, is something that is insecure, and therefore worthy of fear. And to be in a place that is devoid of this painful cycle, is inherently secure. Not only secure, but it is also not 'unknown', because no matter how long we have been addicted to something, there was for everyone a time before this process began, when we stood on level ground, and we were not cast about in a cycle of desire and loss. This is not unknown, because it is where we come from. It may feel like the cold of an unknown future, but it is actually the warm pastures of our homeland from whence we came and to which we can and shall return.

So, to summarise:

The security blanket is not the place we occupy when we are addicted, it is the place we will return to when we get over the addiction. We feel it during the addiction, and misassign it to the thing we are addicted to, because we are familiar with it as a state of mind, because it is where we come from, and where we need to return to. It is always latent within us, but while we are addicted, we block our real access to it, by mistakenly attaching it to something transitory, on which we can never really depend.

The source of the security blanket is not the thing to which we are attached, it is the stable ground we will stand on when we have left this thing behind us. The fear state is not where we will end up when we overcome the addiction, it is the place we are actually living, within the addicted state.

Real security is being safe from lesser inclinations within you. You make your own choices. You are fundamentally in control of your life.

Your material existence is a reflection of your inner existence, so if you exist in a state of inner conflict, then that state will filter into everything you do. You are only one single conscious being. It is not as though there is one person who is trapped within nicotine addiction and another one who makes all the daily decisions, which determine how your life develops. It is the same person.

If you are failing to resolve something fundamental in yourself, then that is the state of consciousness that you are occupying. You are living your life with the lack of control of someone who is injuring themselves for no reason. Everything you do is done through the medium of this state of consciousness.

This is about your relationship with yourself.

This is about your basic capacity to assimilate new information, and form new behavioural patterns on the basis of that information. The fact that a part of you can see the simplicity of this issue demonstrates that you have in you the capacity to understand. If you feel you understand something even only for an instant, then why shouldn't you understand it permanently? When you glimpse the truth, that is your higher self, coming through. Your higher self is not a smoker, because no one in their right mind, possessed of all the facts, would smoke. All you have to do to transcend nicotine addiction is to decide to be yourself.

It really is just about making a decision based upon the actual facts of the situation. Allow yourself to fully accept that you have made the decision and to embrace the consequences. As you embrace the consequences, you allow them to become real and so you are a non-smoker.

If you really do realise that the facts show that you must obviously stop smoking, then by simply making the decision to stop, you have actually won, no matter how daunting making the change may seem.

If you simply try to stop without being fully informed, then you are fighting a system that has established itself at the heart of your conscious mechanism, and you can never really win. That system, though, cannot stand in the face of the power of truth. To glimpse the truth even for an instant is to light a fire within yourself which will never be extinguished. It is like a time bomb. At some point it will go off. You can decide to detonate it now.

"When anxious thoughts are put aside, doing comes from being."

Zen proverb

23

THE SILVER LINING

"But what a terrible waste of time – so much of my life spent smoking, doing all that damage to myself. I've been smoking so long, it's going to be so hard."

No, nothing has been wasted. That is the beautiful irony of the whole smoking phenomenon.

I am of the opinion that everything happens for a reason, and I can safely say that conquering my nicotine addiction was the single most significant and constructive realisation that I have come to in my life. The benefits that I have reaped I could not hope to calculate.

To finally put your foot down on your miscreant mind is one of the most centring things you can do for yourself. I smoked for many years, and having emerged from the experience now, I can see that all the years I spent smoking were to my conscious self what the turning of the key is to a wind-up clock.

If you do not become fully immersed in something then it is not so easy to understand and rise above it. I am glad that I smoked. I would far rather have smoked and come to understand smoking than never have smoked. Where else would I have gained the insight into my own self-realisational process? Nicotine addiction is the big one: the most addictive substance. To transcend it, therefore, must obviously entail some conscious benefits that you would be hard pressed to gain elsewhere. That is not to say that they are unobtainable elsewhere – I am not saying that everyone should smoke in order to experience giving up! What I mean is that this cloud has a particularly fine silver lining!

"Obstacles don't block the path. They are the path."

Zen proverb

It seems to me that the whole tobacco/nicotine phenomenon is a vast evolutionary lesson, which becomes clear when we raise our perceptual camera to its maximum height. There is a specific conscious process to be mastered within the unravelling of nicotine addiction. We are dealing with what I would call the fundamental principle of attachment, which underpins our relationship with the whole of material reality.

Within the dusky threads of nicotine addiction are woven a far more beautiful image. We are attached to everything in our environment to a lesser or greater degree. In the realisation of the true nature of our relationship to nicotine, we can find a reflection of our relationship to every aspect of our existence. From the moment we are born, we are bonding with things that we enjoy or depend upon, and resisting things that we dislike. As a new-born, between the life-giving nourishment and security of our mother's breast, and the contrasting frustration when this is not available to us, we are already forming an attachment to something that gives us a sense of security, and resistance to something that makes us feel insecure. And so it goes as we move forward through life. We relate to the material world through attachment, whether by excess or by lack. And when attachment moves beyond our control, it becomes an addiction and starts to control us. But always underpinning our lives is this one constant, conscious principle, there from birth, and simply re-shaping itself to accommodate each new experience, positive or negative, falling into and out of balance according to the minutiae of our nature and that of the things to which we become more or less attached.

The resolution of nicotine addiction is a model for mastery of the mind. It seems paradoxical that some of the greatest conscious lessons can be learned from one of the most terrible crimes perpetrated upon humankind by itself, but the fact is undeniable. In the process of coming to understand nicotine addiction, we must learn to think both more logically and clearly, and with a level of detachment from cycles of reactive impulse.

It is the inner contradiction of the addicted existence that leads us to make such a big deal of giving up smoking. We are bound into a framework of self-denial and conflict, which leads us to regard stopping smoking as even more complex than smoking itself. Whilst we smoke, we tend to see smoking as a relatively cut-and-dried thing, and giving up as the challenge. The reality is that once we have brushed the cobwebs from our perception, we find that giving up smoking is as simple as making one very basic decision.

So if you are filled with despair at the thought of all those years you have spent pouring nicotine into yourself, take heart - it has not all been for nothing. Do not indulge the fear that because you have smoked or vaped for a long time, it will be especially hard to stop. To be honest, the longer you have smoked the more spectacular your recovery will be. That is what you are going to do. You are not going to stop smoking; you are going to recover from nicotine addiction. Recover, as in to become well again.

It does not matter how much damage you have already done. From the moment you stop, you will be healing. Just because you have spent years damaging yourself, it does not follow that it is too late to repair the damage.

There is no cause for regret in the completion of this journey. The destination is worthy, and the end more than makes up for the suffering along the way. And oh how we suffer, and struggle! From the moment we start to realise we are addicted to nicotine, we are wrestling with the issue of ridding ourselves of it.

A friend commented to me that "Change often happens when you get bored of inner conflict, not when one 'side' or the other 'wins'. Like stopping smoking; I was so weary of the struggle. It was the struggle I gave up, the smoking just got dropped. And it was the struggle more than the smoking that was doing me in!" Enough struggling! Just think calmly and clearly, and let go.

If you have come to this point and you are still not sure that you have dealt with smoking, do not despair.

As I have said, there is for everyone a single moment of realisation at which point they become a non-smoker. We are all different. I have spoken to people about this for merely minutes, and in a flash they saw it, and never smoked again; other people I spent hours with, discussing at length, but it was months or years of turning it over in their head before they finally grasped it. They did all realise, though, and none of them ever smoked again, and they know that they won't.

My point is, do not abandon hope. The end is in sight, I promise! If you are still unsure, read this book again. Read it slowly and carefully. Make sure that you really understand each point that is being made.

Keep the book on you at all times and open it at random when you have a spare moment - see to which areas your eyes are drawn. Everything you need really is here. It's really very simple, and surprisingly easy. You only have to let yourself off the hook.

There really is nothing difficult to do. What could be better - a huge achievement which requires you to do nothing whatsoever? Simplicity really is the key. It is the addiction that clings desperately to the idea that this is a high-stress issue. It tries to get you all worked up and feeling like it's all too much to handle. There is nothing to handle. Simplify. Look at the facts. See what they tell you. Evaluate smoking anew now, for the first time. Treat it as something you have never encountered before. See it for what it is. It does not deserve the anguish it evokes. It is nothing. It is less than nothing, since it actually has a negative effect as well as lacking anything positive. It is an entirely redundant activity that should be far below the discernment threshold of any reasonably-informed human being.

As an experiment perhaps imagine that you are trying to convince someone to start smoking. Try to think of anything you could say in its favour! I think you'll find yourself at a loss for words and I think that will show you that you do understand.

Welcome yourself to the first day of the rest of your life!

"If not now, when?"

Master Rinzai

THE BEGINNING

www.ingramcontent.com/pod-product-compliance
Ingram Content Group UK Ltd.
Pitfield, Milton Keynes, MK11 3LW, UK
UKHW050321241225
466350UK00004B/41